ANXIETY, DEPRESSION, AND ANGER IN PAIN

ANXIETY, DEPRESSION, AND ANGER IN PAIN

RESEARCH FINDINGS AND CLINICAL OPTIONS

EPHREM FERNANDEZ

Southern Methodist University
and
The University of Texas Southwestern
Medical Center

ADVANCED PSYCHOLOGICAL
RESOURCES, INC.
Dallas, Texas

Published by
Advanced Psychological Resources, Inc.
P.O. Box 140383
Dallas, Texas 75214
www.apr-inc.org

Cataloging-in-Publication Data

Fernandez, Ephrem
Anxiety, Depression, and Anger in Pain
     p.   cm.
Includes bibliographical references and index.
ISBN 0-9723164-0-X
1. Pain--Psychological aspects. 2. Pain--Treatment.
3. Anxiety. 4. Depression--Mental. 5. Anger.
RB127.F4 2002
616/.0472

                          LC 2002094079

Printed in Canada by The University of Toronto Press, Inc.
First Edition

This book is dedicated to Raphael, Rebecca, Greté C., and Pravin

Contents

Preface

This book brings together information on three affective disorders most commonly encountered in the clinical context: anxiety, depression, and anger. Specifically, the focus is on the intersection of pain and each of these three affective conditions. As a general rule, only studies *combining* information on both pain and the respective affective disorder are reviewed here. There is also recognition of the comorbidity among these affective disorders.

Each chapter begins with definitions and conceptualization. Phenomenological descriptions are provided while information on symptomatology is drawn from psychiatric nosology. This is followed by epidemiological data on the affective disorder as it relates to the pain population. Where possible, this is broken down according to the type of pain. The core of this book addresses the types of interactions between pain and affect. These go beyond the usual cause-effect statements to an examination of affect as co-occurrent, predisposing factor, precipitant, aggravating factor, consequence, and perpetuating factor in pain. Additionally, biological and psychosocial mechanisms linking pain and affect are elucidated.

Each chapter on affective disorder also contains two clinically oriented subsections: one is about assessment tools and measurement issues, and the other is on treatment techniques. The affective assessment tools are described with reference to psychometric standards but with special emphasis on the practical issues of test selection and administration. The particular relevance of these tests to pain patients is highlighted. The treatment techniques are described and evaluated mainly in terms of outcome as well as process. Both psychological and pharmacological techniques are included. All critiques and evaluations are empirically grounded but restricted to studies that attempt to link pain to the relevant affective disorder. Articles devoted solely to a particular affective disorder (e.g., depression) or pain per sé, are peripheral if not beyond the scope of this book.

Where a treatment or assessment option appears to be un-developed, some attempt is made to draw suggestions from the general literature on treatment of affective disorders. As will be shown, many of these ideas, though potentially useful, still await adaptation or adoption in the population of pain sufferers.

With more than 800 references and many more citations, the reviews making up this book are extensive, though (inevitably) no claims can be made for exhaustiveness. Predominant among the sources are original research reports published over the last 20 years. However, a few relatively dated articles are included by virtue of their status as classics in the field. Also incorporated is research from different countries of the world because that helps boost the generalizability of findings. For the sake of succinctness and coherence, much of the research reviewed is distilled into summary statements of cited articles which are organized accord-ing to a labyrinth of arguments. Readers are also referred to existing reviews of certain subtopics that border on the main con-tent area of this book. Articles of special significance are described at length especially where the methodology is novel or the findings are far-reaching.

As a whole, this book strives to be conceptually based, empirically driven, and clinically oriented. Conceptually, a new framework is constructed to represent the multifarious and dynamic relationships between pain and affect. Empirically, there is a reliance on published data and a critical evaluation of the weight of evidence for the issues at hand. Both the conceptual and the empirical become the bases for clinical implications in the assessment and treatment of affective disorders in pain sufferers.

By the end of this book, greater clarity and closure should be emerge on several important and interesting issues. Readers may expect to be more informed about the prevalence of anxiety, depression, and anger in the pain population as well as the relative prominence of these affective qualities and their occurrence in diff-erent types of pain syndromes. The emergent picture will also contain inferences about the differences in pain sensitivity as a function of affective quality, the contrasting roles of state versus trait affect, and the underlying mechanisms like diathesis-stress theory. Assessment tips such as how to correct for inflated depression scores in pain patients, how to measure anxiety in a way that is relevant to pain sufferers, and how to minimize demand characteristics in anger reports will add a clinical dimension to the picture. Finally, readers may expect greater understanding of a host of treatment options from the biochemical to the psychosocial e.g., attention-diversion and relaxation techniques for anxiety, anti-depressant medications for depression, and integrative approaches to anger.

Sustainability and excitement in a field of study depend not only on the delivery of answers but also on a steady stream of further questions of interest. In this regard, the present treatise arrives at new answers to old questions while also generating issues for future research. These are pointed out at the end of each chapter as well as in the overall conclusion to the book. Ultimately, the goal here is much the same as that for other scholars and clinicians in this field: to expand and strengthen our knowledge of pain and suffering and to improve our clinical services to the many suffering pain patients.

Acknowledgments

Thanks to Ian Aberle, Bob Skinner, and Cynthia Standfield for technical advice, and to Peter Ianuzzi and Jessica Di Vincenzo of the University of Toronto Press for production wizardry. Special thanks to G. Martin F for editorial guidance, to Chris Bhatti and Lori Cohen for bibliographic and indexing assistance, to Abhinav Garg for troubleshooting, and to Stuart Towery for creative solutions. Appreciation is extended to many colleagues, students, and friends who contributed intellectually or emotionally to my writing. To my family members, I remain grateful for your kind thoughts, words, and actions. Finally, I acknowledge the many patients who have enriched my clinical understanding of pain; may your days grow free of suffering and may your lives be fulfilled.

CHAPTER 1

Pain and Affect: Concepts and Definitions

What is the place of emotion or affect in pain? How is affect distinguished from neurological events as well as psychological processes in pain e.g., perception, cognition, motivation, and behavior? What types of affect are most prominent in people with pain? Do these take the form of emotions or moods or psychiatrically diagnosable affective disorders? How do they interact with pain? What are the mechanisms underlying these interactions? How are these affective phenomena assessed? How are they treated? What general findings arise from past research, what clinical options stand out, and what issues remain in need of further investigation? These are the primary questions addressed in this book. To answer them, it will first be necessary to provide definitions of some important terms and concepts. The following sections will draw from past scholarship on pain and the field of affect science to elucidate important aspects of pain, affect, and related constructs. These aspects are integrated within a visual illustration as shown in Figure 1.

Pain-Related Phenomena

Tissue Damage

In everyday parlance, pain is usually described as a feeling of hurt attributable to an injury or affliction of the body. This is not at odds with the view that dominated medicine for most of the last three centuries -- that pain is an aversive sensation emerging out of neurological signals of tissue damage that have been transmitted

1

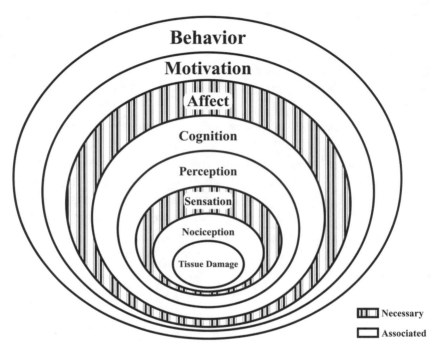

Figure 1. The Pain Experience

from peripheral receptors to a terminal site in the brain. However, there has been ample documentation of tissue damage occurring without pain and pain occurring without tissue damage. To name a few examples, a neurological condition exists in which there is congenital insensitivity to pain, and there are acquired conditions like leprosy and diabetes where tissue damage can occur with no pain; in cancer, metastases and tissue injury can occur long before any pain is felt. Medical ailments aside, many people seem oblivious to injuries sustained in the context of highly engaging or arousing situations like sport or combat. The converse, pain without tissue damage, is evident in chronic pain where the persistence of pain does not indicate ongoing injury, a striking example being phantom limb pain where pain persists in a part of the limb that no longer exists. Tissue damage may be difficult to locate in psychiatric patients who complain of pain, or in circumstances where otherwise healthy individuals have been conditioned to report pain. Given the variety of such examples of the nonequivalence between pain and injury, it is clear that tissue damage cannot be an essential feature of all pain though it may appear to be the origin of pain (Figure 1). At most, it is an associated characteristic (IASP, 1986). This can be taken to mean that its co-occurrence with pain is only probabilistic rather than definitive; it can also be taken to mean that whether there is a basis or not, people (cognitively) associate their pain with tissue damage.

Nociception

Intermediate between the stimulus and the response of pain is a succession of neurological events called nociception (Figure 1). As outlined by Price (1999), this begins with the activation of receptors optimally sensitive to chemical, thermal, or mechanical stimuli which would produce tissue damage immediately or if prolonged. These so-called nociceptors are innervated by primary nociceptive afferent neurons (e.g., A delta and C fibers) which transduce the energy into action potentials that occur at a frequency indicative of the stimulus intensity . Neurotransmitters are released by the nociceptive neurons onto second-order neurons of the dorsal horns of the spinal cord. It is at this site that the critical integration and modulation of signals takes place before transmission along ascending pathways to the brain. The most important of these pathways is the spinothalamic tract with its origin in the dorsal horns of the spinal cord and its destinations in multiple brain sites e.g., reticular formation nuclei of the brainstem and midbrain, superior colliculus, periaqueductal gray, and hypothalamus. The different parts of the cerebral cortex involved in the representation of pain correspond to the different aspects of pain sensation, affect, cognition, and behavior.

Sensation

A sensation is the immediate experience of a physical property of the environment such as color, sound, smell, taste, and touch -- as acquired by the appropriate sense organ of the body. It is the internal representation at the end of the process which began with specialized receptors transducing external energy and generating action potentials in adjacent sensory neurons. Within each sensory modality, the brain encodes sensory information in terms of quality and intensity. Particularly intense or prolonged sensations in a sensory modality can become noxious as when touch becomes pressure and then aching, or when warmth changes into heat and then burning. These may be referred to as nociceptive sensations (Perl, 1980). Unlike somatic sensations, nociceptive sensations may not be restricted in time or space; the painful sensation may spread across the body and its onset and offset may be indistinct. Sensation is a necessary feature of all pain (as illustrated in Figure 1). Without a physical sensation located in some part of the body, pain can only be a metaphor as when people loosely refer to their grief and anguish as painful. However, sensation on its own is not sufficient for pain. As will become clear, other requirements exist.

Perception

Although sensation and perception tend to blend into one process, theoretically, the two are often distinguishable. For one thing, perception is a more active process by which sensory information is organized and interpreted. The sensory information can be selectively attended to, or put into a larger perspective as powerfully demonstrated by the Gestalt psychologist Wertheimer (1923) and by Gibson in his treatise on ecological approaches to visual perception (Gibson, 1979). Thus, the sudden sound of a telephone in a room is instantly recognized and labeled as a ringing sound to which the listener startles or orients. Not until it is put in perspective that this sound is coming from a movie broadcast on the television in the room does the listener realize that there is no cause for further action or alarm. The latter is an illustration of how perception is a more constructive or creative process than its precursor, sensation.

In the same way, nociceptive sensation is accompanied by perception (Figure 1). The same sensation of another person's hand on one's arm is perceived very differently when it is the hand of a friend, the hand of a doctor, or the hand of stranger. The first may be labeled a greeting, the second may be labeled a palpation, and the third may be labeled as a push. These contrasting perceptions are governed not only by the setting but also by the history of one's past experiences of similar sensations. In that sense, perception is more about events than about environmental stimuli.

Cognition

Cognition goes beyond perception (Figure 1). It entails more elaborate and reflective evaluation of information. In addition to encoding, there is storage, transformation, and retrieval of information. As outlined by Ellis and Hunt (1993), the storage of information extends beyond the split-second sensory register to the short-term/working memory of about 20 seconds and long-term memory which can last a lifetime. Other mental processes such as categorization and reasoning are also of interest to cognitive scientists. Of special relevance to cognitive psychopathology are appraisals or the meaning ascribed to events. As reviewed by Stein and Young (1992), such appraisals or interpretations are intimately linked to emotions and affective phenomena. Moreover, they form schemas which are organized bodies of knowledge or conceptual frameworks dictating the kinds of appraisals made by individuals.

Any painful event can be appraised in multifarious ways beyond the causal attributions to tissue damage. These range from implications of danger to interpretations of punishment. With prolonged or repeated experience of pain, the appraisals are likely to develop into schemas that bring about a certain fixity and automaticity of future appraisals. Thus, on the bases of past experiences with acute pain, the chronic pain patient may acquire a faulty schema in which pain is a signal to withdraw or be guarded or take medication -- when in fact the persistence of pain has nothing to do with ongoing tissue damage. It is such schemas and their appraisals that become the targets of intervention in cognitive therapy.

Affect

Closely coupled with each cognitive appraisal is an emotion. This is a subjective feeling grouped along with moods, temperament, and affective disorders under the general category called affect. Though not always apparent, specific cognitions and motivations occur in all affective phenomena (Lazarus, 1991). Such a cognitive-motivational view of affect has become a cornerstone in theories of pain (e.g., Melzack & Casey, 1968; Price & Harkins, 1992; Rollman, 1991).

Various affective phenomena will be elaborated upon later in this chapter. For now, it suffices to say that pain is by definition unpleasant and therefore affective in quality. This makes negative affect a necessary feature of all pain (as illustrated in Figure 1). Affective quality or feeling can range from anger, fear and sadness to guilt, shame, and jealousy -- each associated with a pattern of arousal/activation that motivates the organism to act in ways that are presumably adaptive.

Motivation

Etymologically, motivation comes from the Latin *ex movere* which means "to move out". In psychology, the concept of motivation has evolved along with the study of will (James, 1890), and drive (Freud, 1915; Woodworth, 1918). As outlined by Ferguson (2000), it is now viewed by most psychologists as an internal process that energizes the organism towards a particular action. Whether this energy takes the form of physiological arousal, behavioral mobilization, or something impalpable, it does imply a certain amount or intensity. In addition, there is a directional aspect of motivation that refers to the specific actions the organism tends to (action tendency). Ultimately, the direction and degree of motivation is determined by the individual's momentary emotional state plus dispositional factors like personality, culture, and instinct.

Pain from stepping on hot coals will automatically prompt the average individual to jump off the coals. This may be regarded as an instance of instinctual motivation. However, if the individual's personality leans toward risk-taking, then s/he may be inclined to keep walking. Moreover, if the individual is overcome by the emotion of pride from public admiration of this behavior, then s/he will be motivated to persist in the behavior despite greater pain and risk of tissue damage. Emotional state, therefore, modifies the basic motivational effects exerted by macro-level factors in pain-related behavior.

Behavior

Behavior is the cumulative product of all the foregoing processes (as depicted in Figure 1).   Unlike its precursors (sensation, perception, cognition, and motivation), behavior is observable and may be viewed as a kind of output within a system where the input is some kind of environmental stimulus or event (Skinner, 1953).

In response to injury or noxious stimuli, individuals exhibit stereotypic motor behaviors such as grimacing, subvocalizations (e.g., "ouch"), and withdrawal and other protective reflexes.   More purposive behaviors also occur in the form of extended verbal communication, help-seeking, and changes in daily activities. These are dependent on the specific motivational effects of the prevailing emotions experienced by the individual.   For instance, anger will probably motivate the pain sufferer to aggressive outbursts, anxiety is likely to trigger avoidance behaviors, and depression will probably demotivate the individual from doing much of anything. Additionally, as emphasized by Fordyce (1976), these behaviors are not only the product of their antecedents but susceptible to operant conditioning by their consequences.

Affective Phenomena

To expand on the term affect introduced earlier, we now define various members in this category: emotions, moods, and temperaments.   What is common to these phenomena is the subjective feeling of pleasantness or unpleasantness.   It was pointed out earlier that affect is intimately linked to cognitive appraisals, action tendencies, and physiological arousal, yet different from each of these.   As explained later, affect has a valenced quality that cognition does not have, and it is private unlike motor behavior.   It is not precisely definable in terms of physiological events because of the lack of psychophysiological specificity: some physiological events may be common to different affective types, or they may differ when the feeling states are reportedly similar.

Emotion

Like cognitions, emotions are private events but they are subjective, often described ostensively or by example. Emotions are valenced i.e. they have a pleasant or unpleasant quality. Cognitions in and of themselves do not possess intrinsic pleasantness or unpleasantness. Emotions vary in intensity but cognitions do not, even though the latter may occur with varying degrees of certainty.

The question of how many types of emotions exist has occupied several scholars. Some have differentiated emotions according to cross-linguistic equivalents in the vocabulary of emotion, others have relied on cross-cultural similarities in facial expression, and the rest seem to have classified emotions on the basis of patterns of autonomic activity or central nervous system mediation. However, none of these approaches has produced a comprehensive taxonomy of emotions that is also universal. Far too many disagreements on this issue have led to an abandonment of the question of basic or so-called primary emotions. A new group of scholars (e.g., Scherer, 1994) prefers the term modal emotions which are not fundamental but merely based on the frequency with which certain synchronized changes occur in all organismic subsystems of emotions. Similarly, the demands of clinical practice have drawn attention away from abstract notions of basic emotions to the reality of common emotions -- common not only in terms of their ubiquity and frequency in human experience (Paanksep, 1994) but also with regard to their inclusion in most typologies of emotion (Skiffington, Fernandez, & McFarland, 1998; Smits, De Boeck, Kuppens & van Mechelen, 2002). From this perspective, joy, and certain negative emotions, namely, anger, fear, sadness, shame, guilt, and envy have come to be regarded as the common emotions of clinical interest.

Mood

Whereas emotions are discrete episodes, moods are relatively continuous processes. Emotions tend to rise and fall sharply in intensity thus having a phasic quality, but moods tend to vary within a small margin of intensity over a longer period of time thus taking on a tonic quality. These temporal and intensity differences aside, emotions are quite traceable to specific stimuli, whereas moods tend to be more obscure in their origins. Emotions are more readily attributable to appraisals than are moods. This should not be taken to mean that moods are devoid of appraisals; instead, the appraisals embedded in moods may simply be less accessible to awareness and articulation. Similarly, the factors that maintain and terminate moods are less apparent than those in emotions, thus giving the former a spontaneous and transient quality.

Temperament and Personality

Personality is a construct that includes dispositions to act, feel, or think. A term that is more relevant to affect is temperament which refers to the entire domain of individual differences modulating a person's reactivity to emotional events (Davidson, 1994). In other words, an individual's temperament disposes him/her to experience particular emotions with a high frequency or particular moods for extended periods of time. It may be viewed as a kind of affective style or affective bias. Like personality, temperaments are partly heritable and partly learned, and they crystallize into schemas that govern the appraisal of events.

State Versus Trait Affect

This is a widely used but potentially misleading dichotomy. "State" refers to the momentary feelings reported by an individual at a point in time (e.g., "right now") whereas "trait" refers to a more enduring disposition or proneness to certain feelings. Using the nomenclature in this chapter, state could mean either an emotional episode or an ongoing mood; saying that I am sad right now says nothing about whether this sadness began two days ago or two minutes ago. Trait, on the other hand, is usually assessed by finding out "how often" one feels a particular way. Thus, trait may tap into the frequency or the persistence of an affective experience. If a person admits to feeling angry very often, that could indicate that his/her anger is recurrent or that it is unremitting; in the former case, there is the added uncertainty about whether the anger is dispositional or situational.

Affective Disorder

Based on the definition of psychopathology in the Diagnostic and Statistical Manual of Mental Disorders-IV-TR (American Psychiatric Association, 2000), an affective phenomenon is deemed a disorder when it is intense, frequent, or enduring enough to produce dysfunction or concern/complaint in the person concerned, his/her significant others, responsible parties, or society at large. Thus, anger can turn into an affective disorder if it amplifies into rage which is typically destructive, and if it recurs or persists long enough to become disruptive or incapacitating. In the absence of impairment, angry behavior might nevertheless appear "abnormal" if it occurs in a manner uncharacteristic of most people. This warrants comparisons of individual behavior with statistical representations of modal behavior and it calls for a keen appreciation of sociocultural norms about what is appropriate versus inappropriate.

In principle, any dysfunction due to an emotional aberration qualifies as an affective disturbance. Depression, anxiety, and anger-related disorders are particularly relevant to the pain population in view of the misfortune, threat, and frustration they elicit (Pilowsky, 1988) and the maladaptive responses they produce e.g., anhedonia, avoidance, and destructiveness, respectively. But one should not ignore guilt, shame, envy, and other emotions which, if intensified, prolonged, or recurrent, would produce dysfunction and thereby qualify as affective disorders too.

Unpleasantness, Suffering, Distress

Because pain is an intrinsically aversive experience, the present treatise focuses on emotions of negative valence. All such emotions are grouped under the general term, negative affect or *negaffect* (Fernandez, Clark & Rudick-Davis, 1999). Additionally, the terms suffering, unpleasantness, and distress should be clarified for these are often used interchangeably. The term unpleasantness is reserved for the instant negatively valenced quality of pain; it needs little or no cognitive appraisal. Distress is the affective reaction to pain and is governed by cognitive appraisals that give it further differentiation e.g., guilt, shame, jealousy. Suffering connotes long, drawn-out distress or anguish as commonly found in chronic intractable pain or chronic illness. Like distress, suffering can assume one or more qualities of negative affect except that it also approaches the point of unbearability.

Summary

Looking back over the concepts in this chapter, it should be re-iterated that none by itself is sufficient for pain. A combination of two features is necessary for pain: physical sensation and negative affect. To further distinguish from other unpleasant sensation such as vertigo and nausea, there is an association of pain with tissue damage. This does not mean objective evidence of tissue damage but a cognitive attribution (on the part of the pain sufferer) that the unpleasant sensation is linked to tissue damage.   Other features that are probabilistically associated with pain are nociception, perception, cognition, motivation, and behavior (as illustrated in Figure 1). These layers add much complexity to the experience of pain. It should also be pointed out that though Figure 1 outlines clearly demarcated layers, the boundaries between the phenomena are fluid enough to permit interaction. This interaction can be bi-directional, especially as in the case of affect and pain sensation. It is such interactions that we seek to characterize in the next chapter.

CHAPTER 2

Interactions Between Pain and Affect

Documented ideas about the affective quality of pain can be traced back to the Aristotelian view which put pain outside the senses and within the passions of the soul. Von Frey (1896), recognized affect but considered it a secondary reaction to pain. Beecher (1957) placed affect under the reactive component of pain, as did Hardy, Wolff, and Goodell (1952). Melzack and Casey (1968) referred to an affective-motivational dimension which together with a sensory-discriminative dimension contributed to the intensity of pain. Today, little dispute exists about the inherence of affect in pain, as evident in the formal definition of pain adopted by the International Association for the Study of Pain: "it is unquestionably a sensation in a part or parts of the body but it is also always unpleasant and therefore also an emotional experience (1986, S217).

The more pressing question now is "How does affect interact with pain?" This chapter expounds six primary models of the relationship between pain and affect. Beginning with a correlational model which is viewed as static, five additional relationships between affect and pain are outlined. These five are considered dynamic models in that they represent an active exchange by which one variable exerts some effect or influence on the other. Each relationship is a different temporal ordering of the two variables (as illustrated in Figures 2-7 adapted from Fernandez, 1998b), and that in turn implies a different mechanism by which one variable influences or is influenced by the other. Not only is this a new way to depict the relationships between pain and affect, it also provides a framework for organizing the vast and sometimes chaotic literature on the relationships between pain and affect.

Finally, it presents valuable guideposts for planning and prescribing treatments for pain and suffering.

Pain-Affect Interactions

Affect as Correlate of Pain

Correlation suggests little more than co-occurrence.   Pain is inherently aversive and hence it co-occurs with negative affect (as illustrated in Figure 2).   This component that makes a sensation aversive may be referred to as unpleasantness. It is instantaneous and driven by minimal appraisal, as in the case of other aversive bodily events such as nausea, suffocation, and vertigo.   The unpleasantness that comes with these sensations should be distinguished from the various types of emotional distress accompanying pain after extended cognitive mediation.   Other scholars (e.g., Price, 1999) also see value in such a distinction between the immediate unpleasantness of pain versus pain that involves more reflective evaluation.   In any case, the unpleasantness is concurrent with all pain and closely coupled with the magnitude of the sensory component of pain (Holroyd, Talbot, Holm, Pingel, Lake, & Saper, 1996; Turk, Rudy & Salovey, 1985). However, it should be noted that this unpleasantness is separable from its sensory counterpart under conditions of experimental manipulation or clinical intervention (Fernandez & Turk, 1992; Fernandez & Turk, 1994; Gracely, 1992).

Most epidemiological reports of comorbidity between pain and affective disorders permit little more than statements of co-occurrence. Such reports, as reviewed later in this book, are based primarily on frequency or percentage data that help authenticate the comorbidity of pain and affect. This implies a static relationship between the two. For example, the numerous reports of comorbidity between chronic pain and depression merely

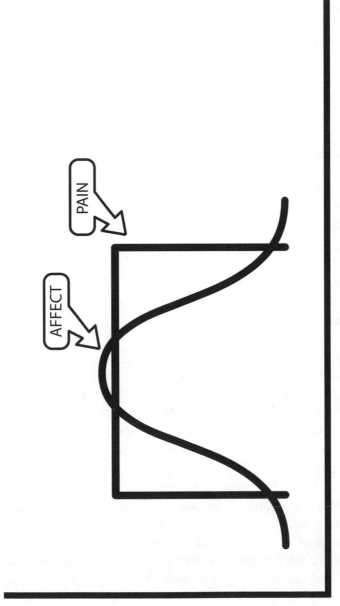

Figure 2: Affect as a correlate of pain.

indicate that where there is chronic pain, there is likely to be depression. Though important in itself, such a discovery does not permit any inference of direction of effects between the variables. It is a far cry from the variety of dynamic interactions that can occur between pain and affect.

Affect as Predisposing Factor in Pain

The first of five dynamic models of pain and affect invokes the concept of predisposition. A predisposing factor is typically an inherent attribute that generates a tendency to a particular outcome. For example, a spherical object is more inclined to roll as compared to a cubic object. The shape of the object is an attribute that governs its likelihood of rolling though shape itself is not proximally responsible for motion. Analogously, biological attributes like skin pigmentation levels can make a person more likely to develop melanoma when exposed to ultraviolet light. Pigmentation as an organismic feature is distal to the melanoma, or alternatively, it is a condition conducive to the emergence of melanoma. In the field of psychosomatics, personality traits are often regarded as predisposing factors for physical ailments. These traits may encapsulate affective qualities (as in the obsessive-compulsive personality, the passive aggressive personality, the depressive personality) that increase the likelihood of a physical problem. For example, it has been hypothesized that certain affective traits render people prone to cancer (Temoshok & Dreher, 1993). There is also suggestion that obsessive-compulsive traits might be predisposing factors in insomnia (Tan, 1984). Likewise, could there be traits that might predispose a person to experience certain stimuli as painful? Figure 3 illustrates such a scenario. As shown, the predisposing affect temporally precedes the pain but in a distal fashion.

Engel's (1959) account of a pain-prone personality was one of the earliest documented examples of how personality traits

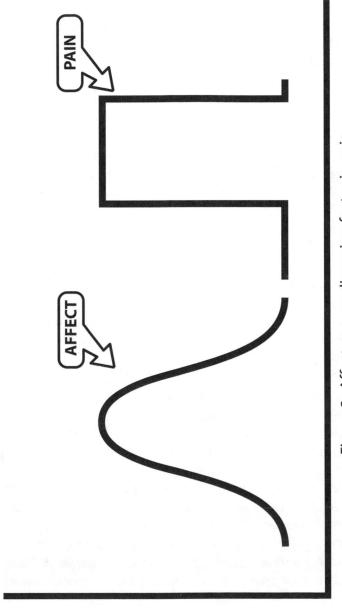

Figure 3: Affect as a predisposing factor in pain.

(centering around guilt) might govern individual differences in pain perception. Similarly, Blumer and Heilbronn (1982) outlined a profile of traits predisposing people to chronic pain. Though the label "psychogenic pain" is now unpopular among pain scholars, the search for dispositional traits in pain patients continues unabated with the aid of various personality assessment tools. This is supported by observations (e.g. Gatchel & Weisberg, 2000) that more than 50% of pain patients in a functional restoration program meet criteria for at least one personality disorder.

Another way in which affect can operate as a distal cause of pain, is through conversion reaction (Ford, 1995). Here, psychological conflicts or past trauma develop into pain and other physical symptoms that often defy pure neurological explanations. The origin of the trauma can range from mental health crises (Chaturvedi & Albert, 1986) to work-related injury (Allodi & Goldstein, 1995). In the case of women with dyspareunia and pelvic pain, a frequent cause is molestation during childhood (Walker, Katon, Harrop-Griffiths et al. 1988; Rapkin, Kames, Darke et al. 1990). The actual delay between trauma and physical symptoms varies, but there is little doubt that post-traumatic stress is generally associated with increased pain (Geisser, Roth, Bachman & Eckert, 1996).

Affect as Precipitating Factor in Pain

In contrast to the distal effects of the predisposing factor, the precipitating factor is a relatively immediate trigger of a response. Using the earlier analogy from physics, the ball that rolls down a slope when pushed, is under the immediate effect of pushing. In other words, the precipitating event is a push, though other distal factors may operate. Similarly, in the psychosomatics of pain, affect can operate as a proximal trigger of pain (as illustrated in Figure 4). As will be discussed at length in Chapter 3, anxiety has a relatively abrupt effect on pain from dental procedures, surgery,

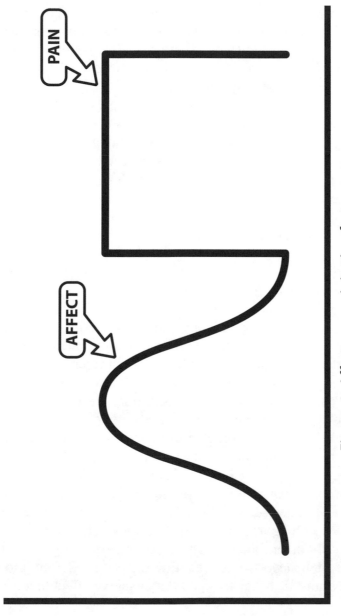

Figure 4: Affect as precipitating factor

and other invasive medical interventions. For example, needle phobics report pain and recoil from the stimulus even before contact between needle and flesh. Moreover, the possibility that preoperative anxiety might produce postoperative pain has been the subject of much interest. There are also numerous reports of panic attacks leading to chest pain, as reviewed in Chapter 3.

The mechanism by which affect actually triggers pain is unlike that of conversion reaction where unresolved conflicts and trauma are somatically communicated. Instead, there is reason to believe that anxiety involves important changes in psychological state. Specifically, anxiety leads to hypervigilance, arousal, and judgmental bias. These increase the likelihood that a stimulus will be perceived as painful.

Affect as Exacerbating Factor in Pain

An exacerbating factor is one that aggravates rather than initiates a response. Returning to the example from physics, a ball that has been pushed downhill might accelerate in speed when a gust of wind blows it along. By analogy, even when it is not the cause of pain, affect may take on the role of aggravating one's existing pain (as illustrated in Figure 5). With origins in interpersonal conflict and non pain-related circumstances, affective distress can still augment pain. Thus, many pain sufferers relate how their pain "flares up" during moments of intense emotion. The mechanism here may be that of physiological reactivity as propounded by Flor, Birbaumer, Schugens and Lutzenberger (1992). Affect is known to produce endocrine changes along with sympathetic nervous system arousal that may have an intensifying effect on ongoing pain. Thus, anger (especially when suppressed) aggravates pain (Kerns, Rosenberg & Jacob, 1994); of course, this is further moderated by other factors such as personality and gender (Burns, Johnson, Mahoney, Devine & Pawl, 1996). In addition, the possibility must be acknowledged that negative affect that is an

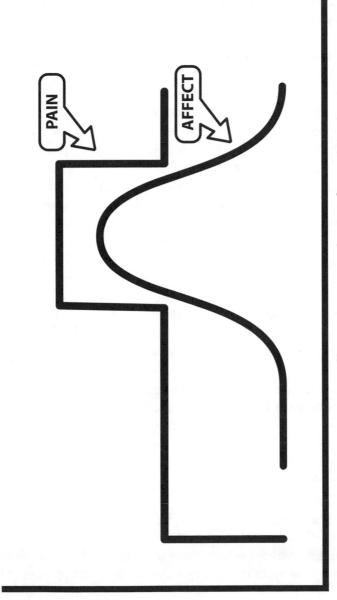

Figure 5: Affect as an exacerbating factor in pain.

offshoot of pain can return to influence that pain, thereby becoming part of a vicious cycle in which affect compounds pain which begets more affective disturbance that further amplifies the pain, and so on.

Affect as Consequence of Pain

A consequence implies temporal accompaniment rather than temporal precedence but furthermore, it implies a causal link between precursor and consequence. Returning to the analogy from physics, the ball rolling downhill may produce its own effect on the terrain that enables rolling. Similarly, pain can generate its own degree of affective distress (as illustrated in Figure 6). At this stage, distress is more than just the basic unpleasantness that is found in all pain. It is now differentiated by complex cognitive mediation into fear, guilt, shame, or any emotion as the case may be. The particular emotion may be stretched out into an enduring mood or, in extreme cases, an affective disorder. Of these, depression has received the overwhelming amount of attention in pain research, anxiety less so, and anger least of all. With regard to depression, the evidence points to a greater role as consequence rather than cause of pain (e.g., Gamsa, 1990). However, this may not apply to other affective types. It should also be clarified that there need not be a proportional relationship between pain and distress. To assert that affective distress is a consequence of pain simply means that it is temporally sequenced after pain, and causally linked to the pain. The latter assumption has not always been evident although new statistical paradigms now permit more rigorous testing of causation.

Affect as Perpetuating Factor in Pain

To perpetuate an event is to extend it in time rather than to amplify it in intensity. Further extending the analogy from physics, the ball

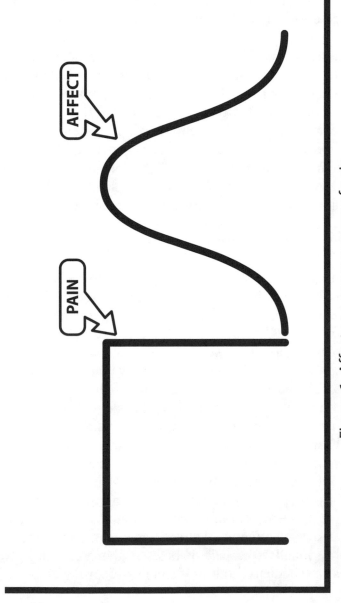

Figure 6: Affect as a consequence of pain.

that was pushed downhill, picked up speed as a wind blew, and continued to roll at a steady pace because of certain features of the terrain that are ideal for rolling. Similarly, certain conditions may be conducive to maintaining pain even if they did not initiate pain (as illustrated in Figure 7). Pain behaviors such as complaining and listlessness may be reinforced by consequences that are pleasing to the pain patient. Various behavior-analytic studies (e.g., Block, Kremer, & Gaylor, 1980; Fernandez & McDowell, 1995) have demonstrated that pain behaviors flourish in a social environment characterized by attention and solicitude which are obviously positive in terms of the affect generated. These pain behaviors may culminate in a sick role that is seemingly characterized by perpetual suffering and disability when in actual fact the patient derives secondary gain and positive affect from this condition. In extreme cases, this may deteriorate into diagnosable disorders such as malingering or factitious disorder (Fernandez, 1998b).

Summarizing with reference to the analogy from physics, a ball rolling downhill is more than the conjunction of an object and an event. The ball rolls as it is inclined to roll by virtue of its spherical properties, because it is pushed, and because its rolling motion is accelerated by a sudden gust. When the gust subsides, the rolling continues because of the available sloping terrain without which the ball would come to a halt. Furthermore, the rolling motion itself may smoothen the slope by getting rid of obstacles and irregularities, thus making it easier to roll. The ball in this scenario is analogous to pain -- which is clearly more than just a correlate of affect. The pain occurs because it is inclined to occur by inherent personality attributes, because it is proximally triggered by affect, and because it is aggravated by affective influences extraneous to pain. Furthermore, the pain produces a certain measure of affective distress which can contribute to even more pain. Finally, the pain persists if the prevailing affective conditions are conducive to it or if a contingency develops in

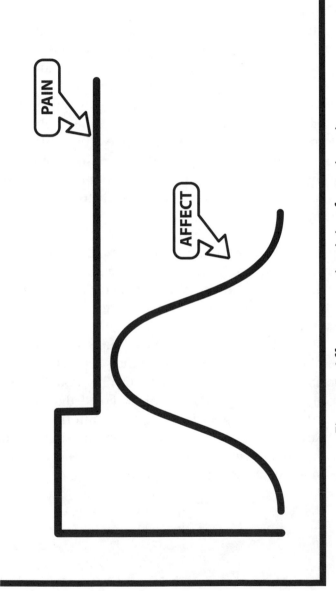

Figure 7: Affect as a maintaining factor in pain.

which affect requires pain. Thus, pain and affect may be more than static co-occurrences, but dynamically related over time. By considering the variety of possible roles of affect as co-occurrent, predisposing factor, precipitant, exacerbating factor, consequence, or perpetuating factor in pain, more sense can be made of the etiology and mechanisms of pain. Treatment options can be better differentiated and tailored to the needs of the pain sufferer. If the objective is to alleviate pain, and affect is the predisposing factor, then characterological change will be an avenue to improvement. On the other hand, affect as a precipitant is more likely to respond to short-term intervention on the affective trigger itself. When affect is an exacerbating factor, it may require focused intervention to diffuse the aggravator in order to reduce the intensity of pain. Affect as a perpetuating factor may call for changes in the environmental conditions maintaining pain.   If affective disturbance is purely a consequence of pain, then affective remediation will do little for the pain sensation. If, however, affect is reciprocally related to pain, then both pain and affect warrant intervention. Finally, if affect is merely a correlate of pain, then it is possible that a third superordinate factor is responsible and therefore warrants intervention.

The new framework presented here will be adopted throughout the next three chapters on anxiety, depression, and anger in pain. In doing so, more order can be brought to this vast literature on affect and pain. It will be noted that the evidence surveyed under each category is not always uniform in quantity or quality.   Nevertheless, by organizing the material within this structure, the complexity of the relationships between pain and affect can be illuminated with greater clarity.

Pain and the Core of Negative Affect

The affective component itself can be further differentiated. It can take the form of instant unpleasantness, distress in the form of negative emotions, or extreme suffering manifested as affective disorders. The negative emotions may range from defensive emotions such as anger, fear, and sadness, to self-conscious emotions such as shame, guilt, and envy. Affective disorders may simply be extreme forms of any of these emotions. We now turn to the question of which emotions or affective disturbances are most prominent in pain.

Aversive situations often generate multiple emotions rather than a single emotional reaction. Victims of crime usually feel hurt or distraught by the violation to one's body or property, rage at the perpetrator, and apprehensiveness about being victimized again. The loss of a loved one is often followed by profound sorrow, but also resentment at being "abandoned", and possible guilt over one's own survival. Failure on an exam often leads to feelings of inadequacy about one's performance, disaffection towards the person making the judgment of failure, and jealousy at others who did not fail. Natural catastrophes too produce a myriad of emotions such as pity for one's hardship, remorse over the failure to predict or avert disaster, fear of recurrence of the disaster, and anger at ill fate. Each of the abovementioned events has several points of focus (e.g., self, others, destiny) that become the subject of multiple appraisals producing multiple emotions.

Pain, being a complex aversive experience, carries many implications for the individual experiencing it. The person in pain may be irritated by its nagging quality, terrified by occasional spikes of intense pain, confused about the underlying cause, frustrated by treatment failures, and demoralized by his/her decline in mobility and physical functioning. Therefore, it is most likely that there will be more than one monolithic emotion experienced by these pain patients.

Research and clinical anecdotes seem to concur that anxiety, depression, and anger are the three main affective presentations in pain patients. These syndromes are extensions of the discrete emotions of fear, sadness, and anger, respectively. They appear in virtually every typology of primary emotions, and are encountered widely in clinical settings. In the pain population, they are especially prevalent and have become the thrust of most research on affective disturbance in pain. Therefore, anxiety, depression, and anger disorders (or their counterparts of fear, sadness, and anger) may be collectively labeled as the core of negative affect.

Across several studies of pain patients, anxiety, depression, and anger have appeared under a common umbrella (Bandell-Hockstra, Abu-Saad, Passchier & Knipschild, 1999; Elliott & Harkins, 1992; Glover, Dibble, Dodd, & Miaskowski, 1995; Kristjansdottir, 1997; Rugh, Hatch, Moore, Cyr-Provost, Boutros & Pellegrino, 1990). Conceptually, theses affective types seem to be recognized as central to the pain experience.

Some empirical research has sought to determine the relative salience of the above affective types as compared to other emotions in pain populations. Fernandez and Milburn (1994) obtained visual analogue ratings of 10 emotions (making up Izard's 1991 taxonomy of emotions) as experienced by 40 inpatients with chronic pain. These patients reported moderate to high levels of anger, fear, and sadness, moderate to low levels of guilt, shame, disgust, and contempt, and minimal levels of joy, surprise, and interest. Understandably, positive affect was relatively inconspicuous in the self-report of this sample whereas negative emotions prevailed. What is highly pertinent is that of the negative emotions, a subset comprising anger, fear, and sadness accounted for the bulk of the variance in the affective component of pain.

Focusing solely on the negative spectrum of emotion in chronic pain patients, Fernandez, Clark and Rudick-Davis (1999) attempted to separate affect due to pain from other sources of negative affect.   A survey was undertaken of 110 chronic pain patients presenting at a pain clinic. Patients voluntarily answered six questions about anger, fear, sadness, shame, guilt, and envy. They provided a 0-10 point rating of how often they had experienced each of the six emotions over the preceding 30 days, 0 designating *never*, and 10 designating *always*; in addition, they made an attribution of the degree to which each affective state was due to pain using a 10-point scale anchored at 0 for *not at all* and 10 for *totally*. Results revealed that anger was the most dominant emotion, occupying patients about 70% of the time, and two-thirds of it was attributed to pain itself. Next was fear, and then sadness which prevailed about 60% of the time. Beyond that, there was a marked drop in ratings for shame, guilt, and envy which occurred about 40% of the time and were primarily due to non pain-related factors. Inferential tests confirmed the dominance of anger, fear, and sadness over other negative emotions in chronic pain and their close relationship with pain rather than extraneous factors.

Clinically too, anxiety, depression and anger have attained a special status in the chronic pain population. One of the most common diagnoses given to pain patients in the 1980's was "Adjustment Disorder with Mixed Emotional Features", a label found in DSM-III (American Psychiatric Association, 1980). The primary features of this subtype were anxiety and depression but it was also applicable to anger as an emotional component. This adds further support to the idea that anxiety, depression, and anger are the most salient features in the affective profile of pain patients. Mayou and Hawton (1986) had expressed a similar view that the most common affective disorder in the medically ill is an undifferentiated neurotic pattern with symptoms of anxiety and depression.   Even though Adjustment Disorder with Mixed Emotional Features does not exist as a separate diagnosis in DSM-IV-TR (American Psychiatric Association, 2000), there are comparable diagnostic labels for the frequent combination of anxiety, depression, and anger in pain patients. Foremost among these is Adjustment Disorder with Mixed Disturbance of Emotions and Conduct. This embraces all the affective reactions to a stressor such as painful injury, and it allows for the inclusion of aggressive and other behaviors consistent with underlying feelings of anger.

The evolving idea of a core of negative affect is also consistent with epidemiological findings. Due to the unavailability of diagnostic labels for anger, less has been made of this emotion until recent references to a comorbidity between anger and anxiety (e.g., Suinn, 2001) or anger and depression (Goodyer & Cooper, 1993). However, the idea of comorbidity between anxiety and depression has had a long history. Abraham (1911) was among the first to note that depression was as prevalent as anxiety in neurosis and psychosis. He remarked "The two affects are often present together or successively in one individual; so that a patient suffering from an anxiety-neurosis will be subject to states of mental depression, and a melancholic will complain of having anxiety" (Abraham, 1924, p.418). Today, DSM-IV-TR (American Psychiatric Association, 2000) lists an adjustment disorder with mixed anxiety and depressed mood. This refers to a combination of depressive and anxious responding (to a stressor) that exceeds what is expected or leads to significant impairment. DSM-IV-TR further recognizes the need for more study of a mixed anxiety-depressive disorder. This diagnostic label is used to refer to dysphoric mood lasting for a period of at least one month. In addition, there is a four-week minimum during which at least four of the following symptoms must occur: difficulties with memory or concentration, sleep disturbance, fatigue or low energy, irritability, worrying, being easily moved to tears, hypervigilance, anticipating the worst, hopelessness, and worthlessness or low self-esteem. Even though the abovementioned diagnostic label does not make reference to "anger" as such, there are features of anxiety, depression, and anger that are embedded in it. This is consistent with the notion of a core of negative affect in psychiatric nosology.

Summary

This chapter has explained how affect is not merely a static correlate of pain but a dynamic partner in pain. It can predispose, precipitate, aggravate, accompany, or perpetuate pain. The most common types of this affect in pain sufferers are anxiety, depression, and anger, which are derivatives of the fundamental emotions of fear, sadness, and anger. These have special evolutionary significance because they correspond to the basic flight/fight/yield repertoire in the face of aversive stimuli.

CHAPTER 3

Anxiety and Pain

Definition and Conceptualization

Where there is pain, there is almost invariably an element of fear motivating the organism to the defensive response of escape or avoidance. When that subjective feeling of fear occurs together with cognitive, behavioral, and physiological features, it produces an affective complex known as anxiety. Like pain, anxiety can be realistic or unrealistic; the latter has been referred to as neurotic anxiety. If it significantly impairs everyday functioning (e.g., occupational, social), it becomes an anxiety disorder.

As classified in DSM-IV-TR (American Psychiatric Association, 2000), a dozen anxiety disorders exist: agoraphobia, panic disorder with agoraphobia, panic disorder without agoraphobia, agoraphobia without history of panic disorder, specific phobia, social phobia, obsessive compulsive disorder, posttraumatic stress disorder, acute stress disorder, generalized anxiety disorder, anxiety disorder due to a general medical condition, and substance-induced anxiety disorder. For prominent anxiety or phobic avoidance that does not fit into the above types, a miscellaneous diagnosis is used: anxiety disorder not otherwise specified.

Of the above anxiety disorders, specific phobia has special relevance to pain. This refers to persistently intense fear and avoidance of a circumscribed object or situation. Pain or the prospect of pain can be a powerful trigger of anxiety in patients undergoing surgery and other invasive procedures. Pre-surgical anxiety (which can reach phobic proportions) is a great concern because it may hinder receptiveness to treatment and the recovery process following treatment. A variation of this problem is blood-injury phobia in which the intense apprehension and fear of injections and minor medical procedures leads to avoidance of such procedures and related stimuli.

Panic Disorder is characterized by a pattern of panic attacks or sudden feelings of intense fear, terror, or loss of control. These feelings co-occur with somatic symptoms such as shortness of breath, palpitations, dizziness, trembling, shaking, and paresthesias. It used to be assumed that such attacks are mysterious or spontaneous events but critical evaluation has revealed that just because individuals do not recognize the situational triggers of their panic does not mean that the panic is random or uncued (Rapee, 1993). The panic may be related to underlying fear of dying, fainting, going crazy, or having a heart attack. The last of these is often the case in patients with non-specific chest pain. This pain rarely points to cardiac disease but recurs often enough to warrant special attention to this group of pain patients.

Generalized anxiety disorder may exist in chronic pain sufferers. This takes the form of pervasive rumination or worry about a variety of situations involving pain e.g., recreational activities, household chores, social events and occupational tasks. According to Rapee (1991), it may also be a premorbid trait – in this case, existing prior to the onset of the pain.

Finally, there is the risk of posttraumatic stress disorder in the pain population. Not only is this characterized by marked fear and avoidance, but also by a tendency to hypervigilance, increased physiological arousal, and re-experiencing of the traumatic event. Typically, the traumatic stimulus is an encounter with actual or threatened injury of a serious nature. Because chronic pain is often the result of traumatic injury, it introduces a likelihood of posttraumatic distress. However, this particular anxiety disorder has not yet attracted sufficient attention from pain researchers.

To appreciate the role of fear in pain, one might turn to the psychology of emotions. The root of an emotion is in cognition. In the case of fear or anxiety, this is usually a judgment of danger or vulnerability or a set of such appraisals forming a schema for processing information. Such cognitive appraisals give rise to fear which varies in intensity from mere worry to panic or terror. This in turn generates action tendencies (Frijda, 1986) or motivations to specific behaviors of adaptive value e.g., withdrawal, escape, avoidance. On the whole, this view of emotions as cognitively driven and motivationally oriented has received compelling support from both theory and empirical research on the psychology of emotions (Buck, 1985; Lazarus, 1991).

Therefore, in the present context, one question that arises is "What cognitions about pain are responsible for anxiety?" Put another way, "What are pain patients anxious about?" The reasons are manifold but some of the stock answers are:

1. pain itself
2. pain connotes danger of damage, disfigurement, disability, or even death
3. pain may recur or not go away
4. pain may intensify or get worse
5. pain may interfere with sleep or other routines
6. pain may become a social stigma
7. pain may be disempowering
8. fear of anxiety itself

The first object of anxiety is the pain itself. This makes sense because pain is intrinsically and invariably aversive. Fear of pain has been acknowledged in the case of pelvic pain (Millstein et al. 1984) and dental pain (Wardle, 1982) to cite a few examples. Moreover, pain signals danger. Fear implies perceived threat and pain is a sophisticated warning system of threats to the body. It can signal actual injury, disfigurement, loss of function, or even impending death. As with many cognitive precursors of emotion, these interpretations of danger may lie beneath awareness, yet their contribution to fear and anxiety is veritable. Compounding the perceived dangers are thoughts about the intensification or prolongation of pain. People may be able to withstand mild, momentary pain but the prospect of eternal pain or escalation of pain over time can be terrifying to those whose coping resources are already stretched. Often it is the impact of pain on various activities that is dreaded; these include interference with basic physical functions such as sleep and sexual activity as well as recreational activities such as sport and traveling. Those in intractable pain also voice fears of personal disempowerment and social stigmatization. Finally, one object of fear may be the anxiety itself. Asmundson et al. (1998) refers to this as anxiety sensitivity which includes a fear of somatic symptoms and fear of cognitive and emotional dyscontrol.

Axiomatic as the connection is between perceived danger and fear, so is the link between fear and motivation to escape or avoid the feared stimulus. These so-called action tendencies are regarded as the essence of the emotion (Frijda, 1986). From the action tendencies, proceeds action. The action may indeed take the form of escape and avoidance from painful activity (Cipher & Fernandez, 1997) or from work and other obligations (Waddell, Newton, Henderson, Somerville & Main, 1993). These behaviors are the end points in the process of adaptation to the emotional stimulus.

Although fear is embedded in all anxiety, it merits further elaboration. For one thing, anxiety tends to be tonic instead of phasic. This makes it more like a mood than a discrete emotion. In fact, the term anxiety actually entered the psychological literature by way of translation of Freud's "angst" which referred to a combination of negative affect and physiological arousal. The frequent patterns of physiological arousal associated with anxiety are SNS overactivity, increased muscular tension, constriction in the chest, shallow breathing and hyperventilation, heart palpitations, and even dizziness. Also evident are gastrointestinal symptoms such as dry mouth, difficulty swallowing, epigastric discomfort, and even diarrhea. Genitourinary reactions include urgency of urination, impotence in men, and menstrual discomfort in women. These symptoms are important to recognize because they are often subject to misinterpretation by the patient and may add to the pain and overall distress. Anxiety, then, is best described as a construct of several features (Munafo, 1998) including physiological reactions but its central feature remains the emotion of fear.

Epidemiology

It is hardly surprising that pain triggers fear or anxiety in most people by virtue of its threat to survival. The basic epidemiological question to begin with is "what percentage of those in pain experience anxiety disorders?" or alternatively, "what is the prevalence of anxiety disorders in the pain population?" Large (1986) diagnosed anxiety disorders in 8% of a sample of 50 chronic pain patients, as compared to the 25% lifetime prevalence of anxiety disorders in the general population (Kessler et al. 1994). The lifetime prevalence of anxiety disorders in the pain population is not known but is probably much higher than 8%; it is also likely that if subclinical levels of anxiety were included, the prevalence rates would be substantially higher than those reported for diagnosed anxiety disorders alone.

Specific prevalence data for different types of anxiety by gender of pain patients has been reported by Fishbain, Goldberg, Meagher, Steele, and Rosomoff (1986). They obtained psychiatric diagnoses for 283 chronic pain patients consecutively admitted to the Comprehensive Pain Center of the University of Miami. During a three-day period of evaluation by multidisciplinary staff, patients underwent a two-hour semistructured psychiatric interview by a senior psychiatrist in order to determine DSM-III diagnoses. The results are shown in Table 1 which is adapted from Fishbain et al. (1986).

Table 1

Prevalence of Anxiety Disorders in Pain Patients (Based on Fishbain et al. 1986)

Diagnosis	Males (N=156) %	Females (N=127) %	Total (N=283) %
Agoraphobia with panic attacks and simple phobia	1.2	3.2	2.1
Generalized Anxiety Disorder	15.4	15.0	15.2
Obsessive Compulsive Disorder	0.6	1.6	1.1
Post-traumatic stress disorder acute and chronic	1.2	0.8	1.1
Adjustment disorder with anxious mood	40.4	45.7	42.8
Total number of patients with anxiety (anxiety disorders and adjustment disorder with anxious mood)	58.8 **	66.3 **	62.5

** statistically significant difference, p< .01

As shown, adjustment disorder aside, the most prevalent anxiety disorder in chronic pain was generalized anxiety disorder; this was evident in about 15% of patients, regardless of gender. Next in prevalence was agoraphobia with panic attacks and simple phobia – at about 2%. If adjustment disorder with anxious mood is added to the mix, the average prevalence of clinical anxiety in the chronic pain population reaches about 60%. Significantly more females than males have clinical anxiety but this disparity is not as great as that observed for depression (see Chapter 4).

Anxiety by Type of Pain

There is a plethora of epidemiological data pertaining to the subcategories of pain and anxiety. Using a two-stage screening process, Asmundson et al. (1996) found that 26 out of 146 disabled workers with chronic musculoskeletal pain met DSM IV criteria for a current anxiety disorder; of these, 16 were diagnosed with social phobia. Lee, Giles and Drummond (1993) found more anxiety (and depression) in whiplash-injured patients as compared to those without chronic pain. Elevated levels of state anxiety were reported in both acute and chronic low back pain patients, the latter also evidencing mild depression (Ackerman & Stevens, 1989).

Anxiety in Pain of Life-Tthreatening Illnesses

Anxiety has been particularly prevalent in those with chest pain. Since the person experiencing chest pain often views this as a symptom of life-threatening conditions, it is quite understandable that a sense of emergency or even outright panic sets in. Worthington et al. (1997) studied a pool of 1254 emergency ward patients presenting with chest pain as the chief complaint and found that a random sample of 44 revealed high rates of panic disorder. Beitman et al. (1987) found that of 30 atypical or nonanginal chest pain patients, 13 were positive for panic disorder. Graulich et al. (1975) found anxiety higher in those with angina than those without thoracic pain. Conversely, those with anxiety disorders are likely to complain of pain; for example, 24 out of 50 patients with generalized anxiety disorder reported a history of chest pain (Carter & Maddock, 1992).

Cancer pain often brings on anxiety especially when the pain is construed as a sign of disease progression. As Turk and Fernandez (1990) explain, such misinterpretation may turn into symptom preoccupation so that the slightest increase in pain is sensed and interpreted as tumor development. Heim & Oei (1993) found that in a sample of 47 ambulatory male outpatients with prostate cancer, those with pain were significantly more anxious (or depressed) than those without pain. Yet, the pain of cancer is not necessarily more anxiety-provoking than other types of pain. Westwell & Johnson (1988) found higher pain intensity and anxiety among nonmalignant pain disorders than malignant pain disorders. This may be due to the differences in pain levels as well as treatment provided: certain types of neoplastic disease such as lymphoma and even lung cancer are not associated with high levels of pain (Ahles, Ruckdeschel & Blanchard, 1984; Turnbull, 1979) but because of the label "cancer", they are met with great urgency and efforts on the part of health care providers. In this way, the anxiety associated with cancer may be less due to the direct effects of pain than to preconceived ideas about disfigurement and death that are attributed to this disease.

Anxiety in Other Painful Clinical Conditions

Anxiety has been evident also among those with chronic, post-herpetic pain (Dworkin et al., 1992), those with a long history of menstrual pain (Salter, 1985), headache inpatients (Villarreal, 1995) and fibromyalgia sufferers (Krag et al. 1994). Twenty percent of psychiatric patients with chronic pain also experience anxiety Chaturvedi (1986).

Anxiety in Experimental Pain

In sharp contrast to these types of clinical pain, experimentally induced pain is relatively free of anxiety as observed long ago by Beecher (1959). Thus Chapman, Dingman and Ginzberg (1965) showed that systemic analgesics normally relieving clinical pain did not alter pain induced by a radiant heat source. This is explainable by subjects interpretations of the laboratory context: most participants in pain experiments assume that in the controlled environment of a laboratory, pain will not cause tissue damage, that it will not last indefinitely, and that one has the freedom to withdraw from the experiment at any time. These beliefs tend to be consistent with the instructions given by the experimenter. Such realistic interpretations tend to make the pain anxiety-free and, in doing so, limit its clinical validity. At the same time, they also highlight the importance of cognitive appraisals in anxiety associated with pain, and thus offer clues to the alleviation of clinical pain.

Is Anxiety Ubiquitous?

Anxiety is obviously not confined to those in pain. This raises the question of its comparative status across subsets of individuals. Hodges, Kline, Barbero and Woodruff (1985) assessed anxiety in children with recurrent abdominal pain (RAP), behaviorally-disordered children (BD), healthy children, and their parents. Results showed that children with RAP reported more anxiety than healthy children, but so did BD children *and* the mothers of both RAP and BD kids. This implies that as prevalent as anxiety is among those with pain, it is certainly not unique to them; groups with contrasting diagnoses may also experience anxiety as long as a distinct set of cognitive precursors is satisfied. Similarly, children of mothers with chronic pain were found to have higher levels of anxiety and depression than children of mothers with diabetes or no illness but other family members of women in chronic pain were also similarly affected (Dura & Beck, 1988).

There are countless studies that report anxiety in various ailments other than pain; these range from neurological conditions (e.g., Parkinsonism, epilepsy, Alzheimer's disease) to respiratory and cerebrovascular diseases. Almost wherever it is probed, anxiety is found to some degree. In fact, existential philosophers and psychologists have long viewed anxiety as part and parcel of the human condition -- hence, the term "existential anxiety" which alludes to the ubiquity of anxiety in human life. What remains to be demonstrated is the *relative* prevalence of anxiety across different conditions or states of being.

Comorbidity

It is also an epidemiological fact that anxiety seldom occurs in isolation from other affective states. Research has repeatedly shown that where there is anxiety there tends to be depression (e.g., Lovibond, & Lovibond, 1995). This co-occurrence is evident in the pain population too. For example, Levenson et al. (1986-7) reported that pain, anxiety, and depression co-occurred in a sample of 80 general medical inpatients. Symptoms of anxiety were more common in a subgroup of 57 chronic pain patients diagnosed with depressive disorder than those without such diagnoses (Krishnan et al. 1985). Becker et al. (1997) found 58% of chronic nonmalignant pain patients seen at a multidisciplinary pain center to have anxiety or depressive disorder. Von Korff et al. (1988) surveyed more than 1000 enrollees of a health maintenance organization and found those with pain had higher levels of both anxiety and depression. Kurtze, Gundersen and Svebak (1998) referred to a striking collinearity between anxiety and depression scores in fibromyalgia patients.

Clearly, there is a comorbidity of anxiety and depression in pain sufferers. This is important because it widens the scope of affective disturbance in this population. Furthermore, it raises the possibility of an interaction between the two types of affect. Along similar lines, there may be a comorbidity of anxiety and anger. Empirical data has been lacking on this issue mainly because research on anger has lagged far behind that on anxiety and depression, (as explained in Chapter 5). Yet, a picture emerges of anger, anxiety, and depression as the most prominent of all affective types found in pain patients and many others. These make up the core of negative affect. Given that, it is likely that these three affective states share an interesting comorbidity that awaits systematic investigation. Such comorbidity should not be taken to mean that anger, anxiety, and depression are more alike than different; rather, it merely suggests that they co-occur and probably interact closely with one another, and they represent the mixed emotions that people routinely experience in response to many events.

Demographic Factors

There has been minimal research on gender differences in the prevalence of anxiety in the pain population. One of the studies that hinges on this issue is by Fowler-Kerry and Lander (1991) who reported that male venipuncture patients were more likely to underestimate pain than their female counterparts. This may be a sign that males were less anxious than females. Epidemiological data on anxiety across different age groups of pain sufferers is also lacking. There are several other sociodemographic variables like ethnicity and socioeconomic status that might also be relevant additions to this list of "yet-to-be-done" research on the epidemiology of anxiety.

Anxiety in Patients With Presumed Pain

Some studies have reported anxiety in situations where pain is not necessarily induced or measured but is implicit. Vassend (1993) for instance found approximately two-thirds of dental patients experiencing pain at least once during a dental visit; between 4.2% and 7.1% experienced high dental anxiety. Millstein et al (1984) found that one of the most common fears during pelvic exam was a fear of pain; one-third of those expecting a pelvic exam had anxiety levels at or higher than that associated with presurgical anxiety.

Significance of Anxiety in Pain Sufferers

Fear, by definition, is an aversive experience and hence it follows that anxiety is unpleasant. Psychologically, this can take varied forms including hypervigilance and worrying. Behaviorally, one of the striking features is escape and avoidance from the feared stimulus. Physiologically, the reactions can be as extreme as hyperventilation, palpitations, and paresthesia.

The autonomic reactions in anxiety are themselves physically uncomfortable to the individual, and are interwoven with other symptoms of illness. It has been shown that physiological symptoms of pain-related anxiety become associated with physical complaints including but not limited to pain (McCracken et al. 1998).

The escape and avoidance behaviors that are associated with anxiety often herald functional impairment. Fear of pain often leads to escape from any situation believed to be pain-causing, and this often includes physical activity. The continued avoidance of such physical activity is responsible for degeneration of the body, and in pain patients this paradoxically leads to even greater sensitivity to pain. Thus, it is no surprise that Crombez et al. (1999) argued that pain-related fear might be more disabling than pain itself, this being evidenced by high correlations between pain-related fear and measures of self-reported disability and behavioral performance.

The psychological features of anxiety are also deleterious to the pain sufferer as are the behavioral and biological aspects. Jones (1985) asserts that the anxiety experienced by chronic pain patients threatens selfhood in relation to life contingencies, self-image and self-actualization, relationships with others, and the sense of psychological and spiritual meaning. At the interpersonal level, one person's anxiety can easily become another person's anxiety. Anxiety places a huge demand for reassurance and support from significant others who are likely to be depleted of their own psychological resources if this demand continues as pain becomes chronic. Moreover, patients themselves deteriorate in terms of self-care and functioning as they become dependent on support from others. Those anxious about pain are also likely to be reluctant to submit to various medical procedures that are necessary but noxious.

Not only does anxiety prognosticate poor adjustment to chronic pain and illness, it is also important in predicting who is likely to respond to treatment. Generally, the research indicates that the greater the anxiety, the poorer the response to treatment. This applies to various types of treatment including cognitive-behavioral intervention, surgery, and physical therapy. For example, nonresponders to TENS were found to exhibit higher anxiety and depression, than did responders (Widerstroem et al. 1992). DeGroot et al. (1997) reported that together with number of analgesics used, gender, and the neurosurgeon's opinion, pre-operative anxiety was associated with poor short-term recovery. For long-term recovery, the predictors were pre-operative anxiety plus fatigue and pain during daily activities. Graver et al. (1995) attempted to predict surgery outcome on the basis of psychological factors in 122 patients with herniated lumbar discs. Less anxiety and fewer psychosomatic symptoms predicted a satisfactory outcome and vice versa.

Some studies remain equivocal about the role of anxiety in predicting treatment responsiveness but this may have something to do with the operationalization of anxiety and other methodological peculiarities. Kreitler et al. (1989) grouped 38 chronic pain patients receiving acupuncture into (i) highly improved, (ii) slightly improved, or (iii) not improved. These groups did not differ according to anxiety measures but only on extraversion scores and variables related to meaning. Jennings et al. (1987) reported that anxiety and locus of control did not relate to satisfaction with care, pain, medications, or complications in 214 patients attending an ambulatory surgery clinic at a U.S. Army medical center. However, these studies are too few in number and limited in generalizability to seriously challenge the general view that anxiety predicts adjustment to pain and response to treatment.

Interactions

As outlined in Chapter 2, there are six primary models to specify the interaction between pain and affect. Anxiety can act as a pre-disposing factor, precipitant, correlate, exacerbating factor, consequence, or perpetuating factor in pain. The literature on anxiety and pain did not evolve within this framework and has been ambiguous with regard to the particular roles played by anxiety in pain. However, it does lend itself to a post-hoc separation of studies according to the abovementioned models. This should bring clarity to the nature of the interaction between pain and anxiety.

Anxiety as a Correlate of Pain

In a sense, the foregoing section on epidemiology exemplifies the first of several models on the role of anxiety in pain: anxiety as a correlate of pain. This is because a prevalence statistic is an index of the proportion of a population with a particular condition at a point in time; in the current context, this proportion is the extent to which anxiety is found in conjunction with pain. Needless to say, there is no suggestion of causality in either direction but only a suggestion of co-occurrence.

Another group of relevant studies is non-epidemiological in nature but directly quantifies the *degree* of correlation between concurrently obtained measures of pain and anxiety. For example, Linton & Goetestam (1985) procured ratings of anxiety, painful muscle tension and reclining time in 16 chronic pain patients over six weeks. They found significant correlations between pain and anxiety and anxiety vs. muscle tension but these correlations were small and sometimes even in the opposite direction. Their general conclusion was that the relationship between pain and anxiety is smaller than previously thought. This weak finding may in turn be related to a methodological shortcoming in the sample size and measures used. On the other hand, Velikova et al. (1995) found significant correlations between pain and anxiety even when the possible mediating influence of illness severity and age were removed. Vassend et al. (1995) reported that anxiety and general somatic complaints were strong correlates of TMD pain. One notable exception involved experimental pain. As previously explained, experimental pain produces limited anxiety; this may well account for the finding that anxiety, neuroticism, extraversion, and sensation-seeking as measured by the Eysenck Personality Inventory (EPI; Eysenck, 1964) and Sensation Seeking Scale (Zuckerman, Kolin, Price & Zoob, 1964) were unrelated to two measures of experimental pain responsivity (Brown, Fader & Barber, 1973).

The majority of correlational studies support the status of anxiety as a correlate of clinical pain. Salter (1985) reported that anxiety correlated with complaints of long-standing painful menstruation. Using multiple regression, Meana, Binik, Khalife and Cohen (1998) found that anxiety and marital adjustment were independent predictors of pain ratings in dyspareunic women. A small positive relationship was reported between anxiety (but not depression) and low back pain (Garron & Leavitt, 1979) while pain behavior during physical exams was significantly associated with self-reported anxiety and depression (Anderson et al. 1992). On the other hand, anxiety (unlike depression) was unrelated to pain frequency, (Kuch et al. 1993). In general, higher patient-perceived pain intensity has been associated with higher anxious symptoms (Varni et al.1996).

Even in some laboratory experiments on pain, certain forms of anxiety and pain have been correlated. For example, cold pressor pain was associated with state anxiety, systolic and diastolic blood pressure (Eller, 1998), and significant relationships emerged between state anxiety and tolerance of ischemic pain (Frid & Singer, 1979). Such a correlated pattern also emerged in an experiment by Bayer et al. (1993) in which subjects (misinformed that an electrical current was being conducted through electrodes to their heads) showed separate but parallel ratings of pain and anxiety.

Anxiety Predisposing Pain

Many studies have considered anxiety as a long-standing trait influencing the perception of pain. Most of these studies have used instruments such as the State-Trait Anxiety Inventory (Spielberger, 1970) or the Manifest Anxiety Scale (Taylor, 1953) to measure trait anxiety and found that people can be predisposed to pain by anxious traits. Early demonstrations of this effect were mainly in the laboratory where pain of electric shock (Schalling & Levander, 1964), experimentally induced finger pain (Morgan & Hortsman, 1978), cold pressor pain (Shiomo, 1978) and pressure pain (Dougher, 1979) were shown to be influenced by trait anxiety. More recently, trait anxiety has been shown to be a predisposing factor in clinical pain too. For example, Chapman and Cox (1977) found that the level of postoperative pain reported by abdominal surgery patients was related to trait anxiety. Bru, Mykeltun and Svebak (1993) found that neck and shoulder pain were also related to trait anxiety and Shocken et al. (1987) observed higher trait anxiety among males with non-cardiac chest pain. Using the 16PF (Cattell, 1965), a strong relationship was found between anxious personality traits and the pain of dysmenorrhea (Hirt & Kurtz, 1967) and thoracic pain (Graulich et al., 1975). Only a small number of studies found little or no effect of trait anxiety on pain perception or behavior (Bruegel, 1971; Johnson, Leventhal & Dabbs, 1971) and these studies focused on postsurgical pain.

There is a need for more studies to directly *compare* trait versus state anxiety in the context of pain. Elton et al. (1978) for instance found that trait anxiety, rather than state anxiety, was correlated with pain tolerance and threshold. However, in the case of chronic pain, the general tendency to be anxious is apparently less predictive of pain than is anxiety over the patient's particular pain sensation (McCracken, Gross, Aikens & Carnrike, 1996). There is also the possibility that trait anxiety itself fuels state anxiety (Wallace, 1987) and it has been posited that trait anxiety may manifest as generalized anxiety across situations (Rapee, 1991).

Someone who is by nature anxious cross-situationally is more likely to be anxious in the state of pain. Research in other areas of clinical psychology does support this link between trait and state in the case of anxiety.

Litt (1996) has offered an explanation of how trait anxiety results in greater pain. Signal detection theory experiments suggest that this effect is largely attributable to an increased response bias rather than enhanced neural sensitivity to pain (Dougher, 1979; Malow et al., 1987). Anxiety also increases vigilance which increases the likelihood of detection and report of pain (Ferguson & Ahles, 1998).

The predisposition to pain is also evident in hypochondriasis which has as one of its primary characteristics, the obsessional fear of illness. Therefore, hypochondriacs have a form of trait anxiety directed to physical symptoms, pain being one. Thus, Pilling, Brannick and Swenson (1967) observed that patients seen in psychiatric consultation had pain symptoms related to anxiety, phobias, and general hypochondriasis. Woodforde and Merskey (1972) found phobias and obsessionality among patients with pain of psychological origin although this was even more so the case among patients with pain of organic basis. Perhaps most striking is the chest pain described by individuals who have an almost hypochondriacal cardiophobia (Eifert, 1992). Other neurotic disorders embodying the trait of anxiety have also been found to predispose individuals to pain (Cormier et al., 1988; Joyce et al., 1986). Using logistic regression, Serlie et al. (1996) found evidence of obsessive compulsiveness, somatization, and psychoneuroticism among patients with noncardiac chest pain. All of these imply a degree of trait anxiety.

Anxiety Precipitating Pain

Whereas the personality trait of anxiety exerts a distal effect on pain, state anxiety tends to be a proximal antecedent of pain. By definition, state anxiety is episodic and its effect on pain is therefore relatively quick. In that sense, it precipitates pain much like a sudden trigger.

Where pain occurs without any sign of organic damage or abnormality, there is an even greater likelihood of psychological precipitants such as anxiety. This is especially apparent in the chest pain literature. Fifty percent of patients with recurrent chest pain (and normal coronary arteries) meet criteria for panic disorder, a condition associated with episodes of unexpected panic attacks without any physiological trigger (Carter, Servan-Schreiber & Perlstein, 1997). This type of chest pain is not the result of cardiovascular disease but a mere result of sudden and extreme anxiety. Similarly, Beitman et al. (1987) reported that of 30 atypical or nonanginal chest pain patients, 13 were positive for panic disorder. Elias et al. (1982) observed that patients with anginal syndrome and no significant coronary artery disease (CAD) had higher levels of anxiety (and depression) than anginal patients with CAD or MI patients. One of the few exceptions to this effect is a study by Bowen, D'Arcy and Orchard (1991) that found no significant difference in panic disorder or self-rated anxiety in patients with chest pain and mitral valve prolapse as compared to patients with chest pain and no cardiac disease.

Where the trigger of chest pain is not a panic attack, there may still be a role for state anxiety. For example, of 50 patients with generalized anxiety disorder, 16 attributed their chest pain to episodes of worry. Cormier et al. (1988) discovered that patients with chest pain but no organic heart disease had significantly higher scores on measures of anxiety, in addition to panic disorder, and simple phobias. They also found that such patients were younger and more likely to be female, a finding corroborated by Channer and Rees (1987).

One interesting paradigm repeatedly used to investigate the acute effects of anxiety on pain links preoperative anxiety with postoperative pain. Preoprerative anxiety is a state of anxiety many patients experience shortly before undergoing surgery. Postoperative pain is the short-term pain lingering after surgery has been completed. The former, so it is generally hypothesized, has a strong influence on the latter. For example, Palermo & Drotar (1996) found that anticipatory anxiety significantly predicted children's postoperative pain. Martelli, Auerbach, Alexander and Mercuri (1987) found that preoperative anxiety was inversely related to adjustment and satisfaction and directly related to pain. Graver et al. (1995) conducted a prospective study in which 122 patients with herniated lumbar discs were assessed before surgery and 12 months postoperatively. The fewer the symptoms of anxiety, the more satisfactory the outcome as measured by several indices including pain behaviors. Taenzer et al. (1986) accounted for half of the variability in postoperative outcome measures by anxiety, extroversion, and depression, but this raises the question about the precise contribution of state anxiety. One answer comes from Reading (1985) who found that anxiety at 32 weeks of pregnancy explained only 5% more of the variance in evaluative scores from the McGill Pain Questionnaire (MPQ; Melzack, 1975) and VAS ratings of pain than was already accounted for by medication use during labor. Boeke, Duivenvorden, Verhage and Zuaveling (1991) found that preoperative anxiety scarcely added to the already negligible prediction of third day postoperative pain by biographical and medical status variables. Further, state anxiety may explain much of the variance in early and active labor pain but not transitional or second stage pain (Lowe, 1987). Other studies (e.g., Johnson et al. 1971; Wallace, 1986) also point to a weak relationship between preoperative anxiety and postoperative pain.

Another interesting paradigm for investigating the relationship between transient or state anxiety and pain involves the experimental induction of anxiety followed by experimentally induced pain. Most of these studies have been conducted by Arntz and colleagues. In two separate investigations, Janssen and Arntz (1996, 1997) induced phobic anxiety by presenting arachnophobics with spiders and then subjecting them to noxious electrical stimulation. Results showed that subjective pain ratings were not influenced by anxiety induced in this fashion. Other studies by Arntz and colleagues (Arntz & De Jong, 1993; Arntz, Dressen &

De Jong, 1994) had obtained similar results. However, this paradigm may be weakened by the use of spider-related anxiety which has no naturalistic connection with electrically induced pain. More appropriately, the relevance of the anxiety to the pain situation has to be considered. Fear of injury and other pain-relevant sources of anxiety may exert a much more powerful effect on pain than would a pain-irrelevant source like spiders. This has been supported by evidence from Dougher, Goldstein and Leight (1987) that anxiety does enhance pain responsivity only when the source of anxiety is related to the pain stimulus. Similarly, Al Absi & Rokke (1991) reported that females made anxious about something irrelevant (potential shock) reported least pain compared to females made anxious about something relevant (cold pressor). Using instructional manipulations of relevant versus irrelevant anxiety, Cornwall (1988) observed that only the former increased electromyographic (EMG) levels and facial grimaces associated with pain.

Other experiments (Bronzo & Powers, 1967; DuRant, Jay, Jerath & Fink, 1988) show that pain does increase with anxiety. More sophisticated designs have permitted near-causal inferences between the two variables of interest. Casten et al. (1995) used path analysis to show that anxiety did predict pain in a geriatric sample. Asmundson and Taylor (1996) employed structural equation modeling to show that anxiety sensitivity does intensify the fear of pain and promote pain-related escape and avoidance.

In summary, the results in this area seem to depend on the research paradigm used. Studies of preoperative anxiety versus postoperative pain show a small association between the two; experiments inducing anxiety and pain in phobics also show little relationship, whereas advanced statistical techniques applied to clinical data seem to provide more support for the notion that anxiety precipitates pain. Other nuances of methodology may further explain the findings in this area. It appears that special attention should be paid to range effects in the study of the effects of state anxiety on pain. Not only is the intensity of the pain a

moderator (Schumacher & Velden, 1984) but also the classification of people into groups of high, medium, and low anxiety
may differentially affect the response to pain (Asmundson &
Norton, 1995).

Anxiety Aggravating Pain

Another role taken on by anxiety in pain is that of an exacerbating
factor. In other words, even when it does not cause pain, anxiety
can aggravate a pre-existing level of pain. Chronic pain offers a
good example in this regard. A person with relatively constant
chronic pain may suddenly enter a phase of anxiety that magnifies
the pain. The anxiety may be related or unrelated to the pain. In
either case, its presence aggravates the pain while its absence
attenuates pain without abolishing it altogether.   There is
insufficient published research on this phenomenon but clinical
anecdotes leave little doubt as to its existence. The same patients
who say that their pain originates in physical factors often speak of
emotional factors like anxiety as responsible for heightening of the
pain; moreover, they state that relaxation does not get rid of the
pain even though it diminishes it. This may be viewed as indirect
evidence for the contribution of anxiety to the aggravation of pain.

Anxiety Perpetuating Pain

Anxiety may modulate not only the intensity but also the duration
of pain. For example, pre-existing pain can become stretched out
in time by anxiety. In one study that deals with this issue, a direct
relationship emerged between postoperative anxiety and the con-
tinuation of postoperative pain over time (Nelson, Zimmerman,
Barnason, Nieven & Schmaderer, 1998).   In the absence of
anxiety, the pain may have been a discrete episode, but in the
presence of anxiety, the pain persists. The mechanism may be one
of operant conditioning if the anxiety triggers helping responses
from significant others thus reinforcing pain. This perpetuating
role of anxiety has not been adequately researched, but anecdotal

evidence does support it. Even though patients tend to be oblivious to this process, clinicians are often acutely aware of how pain reports and behaviors are prolonged by anxiety and the solicitous responses that accompany them. Much research has accumulated on the role of solicitude in maintaining pain but this has rarely been related to the underlying fear on the part of the patient.

Pain Causing Anxiety

Although less common than depression as a consequence of pain, anxiety has been shown to accompany pain. After all, pain is ordinarily a signal of tissue damage. Thus, people who report unremitting dental anxiety have a prior history of significantly more painful and traumatic dental experiences (Davey, 1989). Also, as mentioned earlier, pain may carry other connotations such as disability or in extreme cases, death. For example, prior to diagnosis, 82% of an adolescent sample were afraid that their pain was heart-related but after a diagnosis of costochondritis, 29% continued to worry (Brown & Jamil, 1993). This suggests that the anxiety about pain is driven by the meaning attached to pain (does it pertain to the heart or not?, is it life-threatening or not?). Similarly, Eifert (1992) speaks of cardiophobia in which chest pain is misinterpreted as a heart attack and impending death.

In cancer patients being treated for pain (Strang, 1997), those with higher pain scores expressed significantly more worries about pain progression, fear about the future, and general anxiety about daily living. Fear of pain progression and the future was more pronounced in younger patients and fear of future pain was related to the duration of pain. This latter observation appears consistent with the finding that pain patients with anxiety disorders are more likely to be younger and unemployed (Chaturvedi, 1987). However, a review by Gagliesi & Melzack (1997) claims little evidence for age-related differences in anxiety or depression in chronic pain patients.

Oberle, Paul, Wry and Grace (1990) reported a significant relationship between preoperative pain and postoperative anxiety in elderly patients. There was also a moderate relationship between postoperative pain and postoperative anxiety in all.

Slocumb, Kellner, Rosenfield and Pathak (1989) found significantly more anxiety, depression, hostility, and somatic symptoms in abdominal pain patients than in matched controls attending a gynecology clinic. Hodges et al. (1985) assessed anxiety in children with RAP, behaviorally-disordered children (BD), healthy children, and their parents. Not only was it found that RAP children reported more anxiety than healthy children, but so did BD children *and* the mothers of both RAP and BD kids. This implies that anxiety may be a consequence of pain but it is certainly not confined to those in pain. Different populations of subjects are likely to react with anxiety to different circumstances, though the overriding theme remains an appraisal of danger.

Mechanisms

The question of mechanisms involved in the interaction between pain and anxiety can also be viewed as a question of what other variables mediate these two constructs. Much of this research is speculative, yet there are plausible explanations to be found in psychological and biological processes.

A concomitant of anxiety is the tendency to worry or even catastrophize; this may greatly influence the perception of pain through a process akin to self-fulfilling prophecies. In one early study, less anxious versus more anxious psychiatric patients showed no significant differences in pain tolerance or GSR but psychological responsiveness to pain was greater in the more anxious group which had a tendency to form "anticipatory sets" (Piercy, Elithorn, Pratt & Crosskey, 1955). Such attitudinal bias gathers weight over repeated encounters beginning in childhood (Rollman, 1998). In extreme cases, it culminates in clinical pain disorders like chest pain (Carter & Maddock, 1992).

There is also an attentional component of anxiety that may be part of the mechanism leading to perceived pain. Systematic investigation by Arntz and colleagues has revealed that attention to the noxious stimulus (more so than anxiety) is related to pain impact (Arntz et al. 1991; Arntz et al. 1994; Arntz & de Jong, 1993; Janssen & Arntz, 1996, 1999). However, as pointed out in the earlier section on anxiety as precipitant of pain, the anxiety-provoking stimulus (spiders) in these studies was hardly related to the context of pain (electric shock). When the two are indeed related, attention to pain is often a *derivative* of the anxiety over pain, those who are anxious being inclined to be hypervigilant about the object of their anxiety. This has been demonstrated using the Stroop test which has uncovered anxiety-related attentional bias in chronic pain sufferers (Pincus, Fraser & Pearce, 1998).

To what extent is the anxiety-pain connection mediated by increased sensory discriminability as opposed to increased reporting bias? Roy-Byrne et al. (1985) asserts that panic disorder patients are neither more sensitive to pain (discriminability) nor are they simply more overreactive to pain. However, this issue has been best handled by experiments based on signal detection theory which quantifies discriminability and response bias in terms of two statistical indices, d prime and Beta, respectively. Dougher (1979) for example discovered that trait anxious students undergoing finger pressure stimulation had a lower criterion for reporting painful sensations than did students who were not predisposed to anxiety; however discriminability was no different between these two groups. Malow, West and Sutker (1987) also found that chronic drug abusers who are trait anxious had an increased bias towards reporting pain but reduced discriminability as compared to their nonanxious counterparts from the same population. Using the same pain induction procedure but focusing on state anxiety (induced by the threat of shock), Malow (1981) actually observed decreased discriminability and a lowered tendency to report pain. So, it appears that the effects of anxiety on pain are often mediated by response bias and if anything, decreased discriminability. However, these findings are dependent on a host of methodological factors such as the type of pain induced, the method of assessing anxiety, and the population studied.

There is also a body of research on how anxiety governs the prediction of pain thereby having an impact on perceived pain. Generally, the findings suggest a tendency for anxious individuals to overpredict pain. For instance, under conditions of anxiety or fear, 42 post-addicts tended to overestimate pain intensity (Hill, Flanary, Kornetsky & Wikler, 1952). McCracken, Gross, Sorg and Edmands (1993) found that low back pain patients with greater pain-related anxiety tended to overpredict new pain events, while those with less pain-related anxiety underpredicted their pain; higher predictions of pain, independent of pain reports, were related to less range of motion during painful movement. This overprediction may take several trials before correction. Highly anxious individuals who twice underwent dental treatment expected more pain and anxiety than they experienced and appeared to need more experiences before their predictions became accurate (Arntz, Van Esk & Heijmans, 1990).

Overprediction is also common among children who are still in the process of learning about pain. For example, overestimation of pain was noted in 138 children receiving venipuncture and this was related to anxiety (Lander, Hodgins & Fowler-Kerry, 1992). In 32 girls getting their ears pierced, it was the underprediction of pain for the first ear that led to significantly greater pain when the second ear was pierced (Von Baeyer et al. 1997).

Among the biological factors supposed to mediate anxiety and pain, one of the most common candidates is muscle tension. Although Merskey (1993) has expressed ambivalence about the extent to which pain is worsened by muscle tension resulting from anxiety, evidence has accumulated in favor of the anxiety-muscle tension-pain hypothesis. An earlier-mentioned study by Cornwall (1988) reported EMG increases during pain associated with relevant anxiety. Jensen (1988) found that anxiety-induced muscle spasms are an important mediating mechanism in pain experienced by nonpsychotic psychiatric patients. Flor and colleagues have proposed a detailed psychobiological model of how elevated EMG levels associated with such antecedents as stress and anxiety ultimately produce pain (Flor et al., 1992; Flor & Turk, 1989).

Vascular factors have also been implicated in certain types of pain disorders. In migraine for example, elevations in anxiety four days before migraine (but not on the headache day itself) were associated with increased temporal artery variability three days prior to migraine onset (Feuerstein, Bortolussi, Houle & Labbe, 1983). This was explained in terms of a disregulation theory of migraine relating anxiety to temporal artery change prior to a migraine attack. Blood pressure (BP) may be a mediator between anxiety and pain, numerous experiments showing elevations in BP with anxiety and other experiments showing elevations in BP with pain. One study that attempted to concurrently relate BP to both pain and anxiety was that by Bronzo and Powers (1967) in which pain threshold declined as anxiety went up along with measures of BP and pulse rate. Of course, BP has a certain nonspecificity that links it with emotional arousal in general. Perhaps, it is the affective component of pain that is most increased by BP-related increases in anxiety.

The autonomic correlates of anxiety go beyond blood pressure (Biederman & Schefft, 1994). These same events in the cardiovascular, neurological, and musculoskeletal symptoms may be subject to misinterpretation by already anxious individuals who then become more inclined to report pain.

Other "miscellaneous" biochemical processes have also been summoned to explain the effects of anxiety on pain. Rizzo et al. (1985) mentioned that CNV, a slow cerebral potential, was more marked when pain was accompanied by anxiety. Pancheri et al. (1985) found that state anxiety and subjective pain showed progressive increase during labor but leveled off during final stage of labor; this was paralleled by a similar increase in plasma BE and ACTH from baseline until end of labor. Almay et al. (1978) observed that patients with organic pain syndromes had lower endorphin levels than those with psychogenic pain syndromes but there was no correlation between CSF endorphin levels and degree of anxiety, although CSF endorphin did correlate with depressive symptomatology.

Assessment of Anxiety in Pain Sufferers

Because pain is often viewed as a symptom of a medical ailment, there is a tendency to overlook its affective links, for example the anxiety that may precede or accompany or co-occur with the pain. Even when attending to patients with chest pain and no coronary heart disease, physicians (unless psychiatrically-trained) are not inclined to recognize an anxiety disorder such as panic and even less likely to treat the panic (Carter et al. 1997). Fortunately, psychometric instruments have emerged in the last 50 years to greatly facilitate the quantification and diagnosis of anxiety. These include unidimensional rating scales, standardized questionnaires, behavioral observations, and psychophysiological measures. By far the most common of these is the standardized questionnaire.

The most popular psychometric questionnaire for assessing anxiety across populations including pain sufferers is the STAI or State-Trait Anxiety Inventory (Spielberger, 1970). Its principal contribution to the assessment literature is a distinction between dispositional (trait) versus situational (state) anxiety. This is accomplished by having subjects rate 20 brief statements e.g. "I feel calm" on a 4-point scale ranging from *not at all* to *very much so* with reference to the present moment in time, and then rate a similar set of 20 statements with reference to frequency over time. None of the items pertain to pain as such or (for that matter) any specific situation, but it is conceivable that someone experiencing anxiety due to pain will find the items applicable to that situation. However, Schisler, Lander and Fowler-Kerry (1998) have sharply criticized the use of the STAI in particular two of its forms (C-1 and Y-1) commonly used for assessing trait anxiety and pain in children. Administering these to a sample of 881 hospitalized children revealed insufficient validity and reliability and the need to revise several items of the instrument. While the internal consistency of the STAI may be high, the content validity may be limited by the relative similarity of many of the items. For example, item # 1"I feel calm", #5 "I feel at ease", #8 "I feel rested", #10 "I feel comfortable", #15 "I am relaxed" are almost identical in meaning and so are items 3, 9, 12, 13, 18 which are mere paraphrases of statements about anxiety. While this practice boosts internal consistency, it leaves other important features of anxiety unsampled. There is no reference to action tendencies such as avoidance behavior, minimal reference to cognitive precursors of anxiety such as the perception of threat or the vulnerability of self, and no clear coverage of the physiological correlates that are present in anxiety disorders.

To sample more broadly from the domain of anxiety and to meet the particular need for an anxiety-assessing instrument for people with pain, McCracken, Zayfert and Gross (1992) developed the Pain Anxiety Symptoms Scale (PASS). It attempts to measure the fear of pain in cognitive, behavioral, and physiological terms. In pain patients, this test aids in the prediction of disability. However, Crombez, Vlaeyen, Heuts and Lysens (1999) reported that the PASS was not as effective in this regard as the Fear Avoidance Beliefs Questionairre or FABQ (Waddell et al., 1993), or the Tampa Scale for Kinesiophobia or TSK (Kori, Miller & Todd, 1990). The latter two were superior in predicting self-reported disability and poor behavioral performance, whereas the PASS was more strongly associated with catastrophizing and negative affect. Significant correlations between PASS scores and depression scores also raise questions about the discriminant validity of the instrument within the affective domain.

Perhaps the above problems may also explain some of the factor instability of the PASS. Confirmatory factor analysis has been employed to corroborate the one- and four-factor structures of the PASS in samples of 224 clinic-referred pain patients (Osman, Barrios, Osman & Schneekloth, 1994). Alpha coefficients were high.   However, principal components analysis with oblique rotation partially validated the factorial structure of the PASS with five instead of four factors emerging: catastrophic thoughts, physiological anxiety symptoms, escape/avoidance behaviors, cognitive interference, and coping strategies (Larsen, Taylor & Asmundson, 1997).   Analgesic medication use did not alter the factor solution.   Even though there have been calls for revision of the PASS, it remains more suitable than the STAI for measuring anxiety in pain patients.

Another recent entry to this area has been the Fear of Pain Questionnaire (McNeil & Rainwater, 1998), its most recent version called the FPQ-111 with 30 items and three subscales: severe pain, minor pain, and medical pain.   High scores on this test predict greater escape or avoidance from a pain-relevant behavioral test. McCracken et al. (1996) have found it meaningful to create subsets of anxiety variables by drawing from the Fear of Pain Question-naire, the Fear-Avoidance Beliefs Questionnaire, the PASS, and the trait version of the STAI.

As for other approaches to assessing anxiety in pain suffer-ers, an observational scale for anxiety in children has been developed by Katz (1980) as cited in Shacham and Daut (1981). However, this scale seems to reflect both anxiety and pain. Visual analogue scales have also been used as a matter of convenience. Anxiety is a complex of cognitive, behavioral, and affective com-ponents that are not readily reduced to a unidimensional scale. Ahles et al. (1984) assessed the concurrent validity of VAS meas-ures of anxiety with reference to the STAI and found a lack of agreement between the two.   The individual component of fear within anxiety may be more amenable to unidimensional scaling (e.g., Fernandez, Clark, & Rudick-Davis, 1999), but multiple com-ponents would require multicomponential assessment (e.g., Skiffington, Fernandez & McFarland, 1998).

Treatment of Anxiety in Pain Sufferers

Anxiety has been successfully treated pharmacologically as well as psychologically. This section consists of an account of the many psychological techniques for regulating anxiety along with some exemplary studies of their application to pain patients. Subsequently, there will be a brief survey of the main drugs of choice in the treatment of anxiety.

Psychological Interventions

Psychological intervention is directed at the mind or behavior as the point of entry for changing emotional problems. The techniques are diverse and derive from various schools of psychotherapy. In the context of anxiety in pain patients, the psychological techniques that have been most extensively researched are (i) cognitive strategies such as information-giving, attention-diversion, thought-stopping, and reappraisal, and (ii) behavioral strategies such as self-regulated breathing and muscle relaxation. Miscellaneous methods of relaxation by an external agent have also been used e.g., massage and music. Additionally, complex manipulations such as hypnosis and the enhancement of perceived control have been employed. Finally, there are treatment packages incorporating multiple psychological techniques: these are stress inoculation training and systematic desensitization. The following section reviews research on the applicability of each of these techniques for anxiety management in the pain population.

Information. Anxiety is often rooted in uncertainty and confusion. A student entering an exam without any idea of the content of the examination is likely to become anxious. A patient scheduled for a medical procedure about which s/he has no knowledge of what to expect, is also a candidate for anxiety. Given this feature of the "unknown" in the minds of the anxious, an obvious starting point in the treatment of anxiety is the provision of adequate information. This does not require that every detail be disclosed, for that might overwhelm the patient and backfire with increased anxiety. Rather, "adequate information" means just enough information to address the patient's curiosities and concerns and to allow for informed consent to be granted. Several studies have manipulated information as an independent variable to determine its effects on anxiety and pain.

One clinical situation where information-giving has become a practice is in childbirth and labor pain. This is supported by numerous studies reporting beneficial effects of such information. For example, Klusman (1975) showed that a childbirth education course reduced general anxiety which in turn exerted a significant effect on pain reports during the transition stage of labor.

In general, information prior to surgery diminishes the anxiety about surgery. Informed female patients undergoing minor surgery reported significantly less postoperative pain than noninformed controls (Wallace, 1985). Cholecystectomy patients showed reduced levels of anxiety due to operative pain when they received either information or facilitation (Schwartz-Barcott et al. 1994).

In a systematic study of information-giving relative to other strategies, Wardle (1983) compared four conditions with regard to their effects on anxiety and pain: sensation information, visual distraction, perceived control, or normal practice. The sensation information group showed significantly less anxiety than controls although none of the three treatment conditions differed significantly on anxiety ratings. As for pain, both sensation information and perceived control led to lower ratings than controls.

Many other studies of informational effects on anxiety have been summarized by Gagliano (1988). A primary message emerging from this review of 25 studies is that a video presentation by a role model decreased patients' anxiety, pain, and sympathetic arousal while increasing knowledge, cooperation, and coping ability. However, there was no advantage in terms of long-term retention of knowledge or compliance with medical regimens in video-based education as compared to traditional methods of patient education.

Attention-Diversion. Attention-diversion as used in anxious pain sufferers, ranges along a continuum from passive distraction by external stimuli to active performance of a competing task (Fernandez, 1986). Because attention is finite in capacity, any deployment of its resources to one stimulus/task leaves less available for another. This principle has been utilized in pain sufferers, especially children. Thus, Kuttner (1989) reports case studies of distraction in children by using bubbles and pop-up books, kinesthetic methods (e.g., rocking) and imaginal methods bordering on hypnosis. However, it is unlikely that the effects of attention-diversion on pain are mediated exclusively by alterations of anxious affect; information processing variables must also be relevant.

Pickett & Clum (1982) reported that attention-redirection was more effective than relaxation training, relaxation instructions and no treatment in reducing postsurgical anxiety, although its effect on postoperative pain was equivocal. The pain of childbirth was positively related to anxiety and negatively correlated with self-efficacy, and also negatively correlated with attention distraction and control-predictability coping strategies (Shiloh et al. 1998).

Later research has shown that the benefits of attention-diversion are not unconditional. One important moderating factor is the type of distractor. Wardle (1983) for instance found that visual distraction alone did not significantly reduce anxiety when compared to a control condition. Compared to a hypnotic trance involving a favorite story, behavioral distraction was not as effective in alleviating the anxiety and pain of bone marrow transplants in young children (Kuttner, 1988). Hypnosis does engage attentional mechanisms (Hilgard, 1977; Hilgard & Hilgard, 1975) but a hypnotic trance clearly requires far greater depth of processing and alteration of consciousness than a non-hypnotic distraction task.

Another moderator variable is age of the participant as revealed in a study by Kuttner, Bowman and Teasdale (1988). They randomly assigned 59 children from two age groups (3-6 and 7-20) to 3 conditions: hypnotic imaginative involvement, behavioral distraction, or standard medical practice. Each intervention was repeated. Behavioral distraction produced significant reductions in distress/anxiety only in the older group at second intervention. This might suggest a practice effect in addition to the advantage of age (among children at least) in the response of anxiety to distraction.

In another related study (Smith et al. 1996), an ethnically diverse sample of children with cancer or blood disorders was trained in distraction or hypnosis to reduce pain and anxiety. Predictably, low hypnotizable children did not respond as well as their high hypnotizable counterparts to hypnosis, but they did respond to distraction, which accounted for significant positive effects in distress. In other words, where hypnosis failed, distraction was effective. However, Farthing et al. (1997) compared external distractors (word memory and pursuit-rotor tasks) with internal distractors (guided imagery and suggestions of analgesia) among undergraduate students undergoing cold pressor pain. With regard to pain, none of the experimental treatments was beneficial for low hypnotizable subjects but all of them were effective for high hypnotizable subjects. The different treatment instructions did not affect preimmersion anxiety ratings; therefore, the distraction effects on pain cannot be explained by their effects of anxiety. This raises the strong possibility that even in the absence of anxiety reduction, attention-diversion can block pain perhaps by altering overall awareness of the noxious stimulus.

Awareness of pain may not be completely abolished by distraction. Realistically, an individual may choose to keep a balance between some awareness of the pain and some distraction by non-painful stimuli. This may explain the finding by Muris et al. (1995) that both attending and distracting reduced anxiety in 65% of patients undergoing dental treatment. There may be individual differences in the degree of comfort with distraction, some individuals preferring to track the pain continuously at a low level of awareness or else monitor it intermittently at a higher level of awareness.

Thought-Stopping.   Somewhere between distraction and reappraisal is the technique of thought-stopping. It involves the repetition of a word or phrase in a way that combats absorption with negative thoughts. There is no active attempt to reinterpret the negative, but instead an attempt to interrupt it. This technique has been used for obsessive-compulsive disorder, an anxiety disorder characterized by uncontrollable thoughts that trigger certain dysfunctional behaviors. The success of thought-stopping for obsessional thinking has been limited. Perhaps, it can be put to better use where the thoughts are negative but not obsessional in frequency. Ross (1984) prescribed a thought-stopping procedure for school-age children anticipating a painful diagnostic or treatment intervention. The procedure involved preparing a set of positive statements about the feared event, memorizing them, and then repeating them each time the event comes to mind. This has been used with retarded children as well as short-term acute-care patients and chronically ill children under continuing care.

Thought-stopping is more likely to be used together with other cognitive techniques than on its own. In a case study by Schonfeld (1992), a 55 year-old psychiatric patient was treated for her anxiety, depression, and pain by a combination of thought-stopping, self-talk, and covert assertion. Through a set of five case studies, French & Tupin (1974) illustrated how a mantra (a word or phrase of special personal significance) can be repeated to facilitate a meditative state and combined with relaxation and other adjuncts for managing patient anxiety and pain.

Thought-stopping has a long history in the regulation of negative thoughts including those that trigger anxiety. It seems to have potential as one component in a package for managing anxiety. However, systematic research on this technique in the pain population is yet to be conducted.

Cognitive Reappraisal.   Instead of attempting to abort negative thoughts, greater promise lies in altering them or replacing them with positive alternatives. Also known as self-talk, such cognitive reappraisal lies at the root of cognitive therapy for emotional disturbances (Beck, Emery & Greenberg, 1985; Ellis & Grieger, 1986). This is an obvious treatment option for anxiety. In fact, the cognitive treatment of anxiety is primarily an exercise in reinterpretation, so that anxious persons are trained to identify catastrophizing statements, logically dispute them, seek out evidence against them, and replace them with more realistic (and presumably adaptive) alternatives. The same approach has been used very successfully in the treatment of depression, yet has attracted much less interest in the alleviation of anxiety among those with pain. According to Clark (1986, 1988), panic for example results from the catastrophic misinterpretation of certain bodily sensations. These catastrophic cognitions should therefore be replaced with noncatastrophic alternatives (or what is called decatastrophization).

Two studies illustrate the applicability of cognitive re-appraisal in the present context. Young & Humphrey (1985) assigned hysterectomy patients to a group taught cognitive control over anxiety through a detailed booklet, or a group taught the same skills orally, or an attention-placebo control group. Results showed less pain and distress in both treatment groups as compared to the control group. McCracken (1998) reported that a cognitive mindset characterized by greater acceptance of pain was associated with lower pain intensity reports, less pain-related anxiety, and reduced avoidance.

Reappraisal has been implemented as a key feature of several pain treatment packages (such as stress inoculation -- to be dis-cussed later) and pain management programs. Findings by Boyle and Ciccone (1994) support the use of reappraisal in combination with relaxation for the reduction of anxiety associated with pain. Such a package reduced scores on the tension-anxiety subscale of the POMS in a sample of middle-aged and elderly chronic pain sufferers. In implementing reappraisal, anxiety-provoking statements like "pain means danger", "the pain is unbearable" are disputed and replaced by counterstatements like "hurt does not imply harm", "it is possible to control the pain", respectively. Of course, this is not a matter of simple didactic instruction; rather, it proceeds within an atmosphere of collaborative discovery. The patient might volunteer a particular interpretation of the pain and this is reflected upon by both therapist and patient, evaluated for accuracy, and then retained or replaced with more accurate ideation. A new set of interpretations may not take hold immediately, so it must be reinforced with approval and praise, and further reinforced by reminders at strategic points in time. This invokes the basic principle of shaping that has ben successfully used to modify a variety of behaviors.

Respiratory Regulation. As mentioned at the beginning of this chapter, anxiety is associated with arousal of the sympathetic nervous system, and one of the first physiological functions to be altered is respiration.   Breathing usually becomes shallow and rapid, sometimes reaching the point of hyperventilation (40-60 breaths per minute). This is a common problem in anxiety and panic. Hyperventilation is often responsible for lactic acidosis which in turn makes the individual experience dizziness, sweating, heart palpitations, paresthesia etc (Fried, 1993). Such changes can further compound the individual's perception of anxiety. It follows that the proper regulation of breathing is needed to attenuate anxiety. Breathing to relax entails slowing the pace of breathing, often taking about three seconds to inhale and three seconds to exhale, with a smooth transition from one cycle to the next. This should also be done at the diaphragmatic level instead of the thoracic level, since the former allows maximization of lung capacity for the intake of oxygen. Slow, deep breathing (8-12 breaths per minute) through the nose and using the diaphragm is incompatible with hyperventilation. During an actual panic attack associated with hyperventilation, the patient may breathe into a paper bag so that carbon dioxide collects in the bag and is inhaled thus correcting the excess of oxygen and restoring balance of blood gases.

Typically, the regulation of breathing has been implemented as one of several components in a treatment package, thus making it difficult to isolate its unique contribution to the reduction of anxiety. Nevertheless, the few studies of this technique in pain patients do support its utility. Heitkemper, Layne and Sullivan (1993) found that paced respiration was effective in reducing expected discomfort and STAI scores in children receiving dental care. Zimmermann (1979) showed that respiratory autogenic training was more effective than a traditional psychoprophylactic course in reducing anxiety before labor and reducing pain during labor; expulsion time was also shorter in the respiratory training group than the psychoprophylaxis group. In a case report of a 32-year-old female with anxiety neurosis, headaches and verteborgenous pains, retraining in inhalation and exhalation led to decreased tension of the thoracic muscles that was in turn associated with a decrease in anxiety and the elimination of pain (Svobodova, 1997).

Muscle Relaxation. Breathing and thoracic muscle activity are not the only physiologic features of the anxiety response. In fact, muscle groups in many parts of the body tend to tense up during anxiety. Again, such tension can become a problem in itself, often heightening one's awareness of the anxiety to the point of being overwhelmed and feeling a loss of control over it. Fortunately, the musculoskeletal system is under voluntary control and it is possible for an individual to relax designated muscles of the body. In psychology, this is ordinarily achieved by mere thoughts of muscle relaxation [autogenic relaxation as developed by Schultz (1932)] or by the actions of alternating between flexing and relaxing 16 different muscle groups [progressive muscle relaxation as developed by Jacobson, (1938)]. In practice, these techniques are difficult to separate since bringing a muscle under control behaviorally often entails willing and thinking it through.

In either case, relaxation is antagonistic to muscle tension and engages the parasympathetic nervous system, thus reducing anxiety.

Oest (1987) has reviewed 18 controlled studies on relaxation for anxiety reduction and found strong evidence of its beneficial effects on pain, anxiety and other problems. It should be noted that even though many relaxation exercises produce noticeable changes rather quickly, the benefits are most pronounced with practice. In its original formulation by Jacobson, a course in progressive muscle relaxation could last about three months. However, abbreviated versions (e.g., Paul, 1966) promise proficiency within a few weeks. In a case study of a 20-year-old female patient with temporamandibular dysfunction, (Stam, McGrath & Brooke, 1984), four weekly sessions of relaxation were used to counter anxiety and ultimately eliminate it and the anxiety and pain associated with this condition. Follow-up at 16 months showed maintenance of treatment gains. In another study (Domar et al. 1987), patients scheduled for surgical removal of a skin cancer were required to elicit the relaxation response 20 minutes a day until the day of surgery. These patients reported that relaxation reduced their anxiety several days prior to surgery while control patients who read for 20 minutes a day reported their highest anxiety levels during and after surgery; however, there were no differences in pain perception between the groups.

In contrast to the use of relaxation as a prophylactic method against anxiety, it can also be used as early intervention within a cue-control format. This means that the individual is trained to recognize the problem event (in this case, anxiety) whenever it occurs and regard it as a cue to implement relaxation right away. Such an approach has been prescribed for pain patients (Dolan, Allen & Sawyer, 1982). Another variation of Jacobsonian progressive muscle relaxation has been explored by Carlson & Curran (1994) who refer to stretch-based relaxation training as an alternative to muscle tension release. They have provided a review of the research along with a clinical case example of the effective use of this method for neck pain/tension and anxiety.

Biofeedback-Assisted Relaxation. Voluntary control over muscles can be shaped by greater awareness of the ongoing activity in these muscles.   But, with the exception of very subjective impressions of muscle tension, most people are unable to discern the subtle changes in muscle activity. With the advent of biofeedback about 30 years ago, this barrier was broken as it became possible to receive precise and instantaneous information on many biological processes ordinarily outside the individual's consciousness.   In the case of muscle tension, a person's electromyographic (EMG) activity could be measured and fed back to him or her on a moment-to-moment basis as in the seminal study by Budzynski & Stoyva (1969).   Ever since then, EMG biofeedback has become a tool for facilitating muscle relaxation. Such an approach capitalizes not only on the enhancement of awareness of muscle activity but also helps reify the individual's sense of control over these muscles.   Furthermore, there is an element of operant conditioning by "success feedback" which reinforces change in the desired direction.

To manage anxiety experienced by those in pain, most studies today propose muscle relaxation assisted by biofeedback. Sherman, Gall and Gormly (1979) treated 16 phantom limb patients with progressive muscle relaxation, feedback of muscle tension in the stump and forehead, and reassurance about phantom sensations and their relationship to anxiety. Two of the patients were recent amputees and reported complete relief from pain. At the end of treatment, 8 of the 14 amputees with chronic pain showed almost complete relief from pain, 4 showed significant decreases to a point where they no longer desired treatment, and 2 showed no significant change (both of these possibly driven by secondary gain and failing to learn to relax). Remarkably, treatment effects were maintained at follow-up six months and three years later. Mandke et al. (1996) showed that biofeedback-induced relaxation and behavioral counseling reduced anxiety, pain, and physical symptoms in five patients who underwent coronary artery bypass graft surgery. Bush, Ditto and Feuerstein (1985) found that low back pain patients receiving paraspinal EMG biofeedback showed significant reduction in paraspinal EMG, pain, anxiety, and depression but so did placebo control and no treatment control groups.

The question that arises at this point is whether or not biofeedback-assisted relaxation has an additive effect to relaxation by itself. The data here are less encouraging. Achterberg, Kenner and Casey (1989) found that in multiple fracture patients, relaxation facilitated by EMG biofeedback produced positive effects on state anxiety and discomfort whereas attention and no treatment control conditions produced little change. However, biofeedback was not superior to muscle relaxation by itself. Lobb, Shannon, Rrecer and Allen (1984) randomly assigned 30 females undergoing hysterectomy to (i) relaxation training, biofeedback and desensitization for surgical trauma, (ii) conversations with visiting staff members, or (iii) a control condition. Results were mixed on most variables, the relaxation group witnessing significantly fewer days in postoperative care than the other groups.

The lack of a clear and consistent advantage of biofeedback over relaxation unassisted by biofeedback can probably be explained by differences in participants and procedures. Some participants attach more credibility to biofeedback and the human ability to self-control whereas others are resistant or incredulous. Research on biofeedback has further revealed differential outcomes as a function of modality of feedback and other parameters like duration of feedback training and the muscle site used to generate feedback. These same factors can be exploited to boost the efficacy of biofeedback in the regulation anxiety and tension in pain sufferers.

Touch and Massage. There are occasions when self-regulation of anxiety and tension is not easily accomplished. For some people, the idea of self-regulation holds limited credibility, but for others the difficulty may lie in mastering instructions or adhering to them.   For yet others, the difficulty is one of motivation, or else, the problem may be one of excessive effort or overkill.   In these cases, an external agent of change serves as a better alternative.   Massage falls within this category of relaxation methods where the individual submits to an outside source of change.   The healing effects of touch have long been claimed for many medical conditions -- including pain disorders where physical therapy continues to make an appreciable contribution. Apart from its tension-reducing effects on muscles and its activation of A-β fibers that block pain signals at the spinal gating mechanism, massage works by cortical influences that involve the reduction of anxiety.

In a review of quantitative studies on therapeutic touch published between 1985 and 1995, Spence & Olson (1997) identified 11 studies that collectively demonstrated the beneficial effect of therapeutic touch on pain and anxiety.   More recently, evidence has arisen that children with mild to moderate juvenile arthritis who were massaged by their parents 15 minutes a day for 30 days showed immediate reductions in anxiety and cortisol (stress hormone), and decreases in pain (self-reported, or by report of parents and physicians) over the 30-day period (Field et al. 1997).

Music.   Another external agent for countering anxiety is music.   Though it does not involve the active intervention of an agent upon the individual concerned, it has long been claimed to have everything from relaxing to euphoric effects.   The mechanism goes beyond mere distraction to a veritable change in affect.   Thus, Rodgers (1995) used so-called "anxiolytic music" (without lyrics or singing) to control anxiety of pain pre-, intra- and post-operatively.   In a very painful medical procedure called punch biopsy, Davis (1992) found that patients listening to their choice of music over headphones had significantly lower respiratory rate and overt pain scores than patients in a control condition; however, the generalizability of these findings is questionable for the differences were not significant for colposcopy, cryosurgery, and other procedures.

Hypnosis. Hypnosis has been used in varying forms to reduce the anxiety of several painful conditions. This ranges from the induction of a deep trance by a hypnotherapist to the use of suggestions within a self-regulation format. For children, stories and guided imagery have often been delivered within the framework of hypnosis. On the whole, the results have been encouraging. Hypnosis in the hands of an experienced therapist can be an especially effective tool in the management of anxiety associated with pain.

In a large sample of 52 pediatric surgical patients, Lambert (1996) employed hypnotic suggestions for a favorable post-operative course and found that this led to lower postoperative state anxiety than under control conditions. Most of the pediatric pain patients receiving hypnotherapy have been those with pain linked to cancer or its treatment. In children with leukemia and Non-Hodgkins lymphoma, both direct and indirect suggestions of pain relief yielded significant reductions in pain and anxiety from lumbar punctures (Hawkins, Liossi, Ewart, Hatira & Kosmidis, 1998). Genius' (1995) review of nine systematic studies since 1981 on hypnosis for anxiety, pain, and emesis in child and adolescent cancer patients was equally favorable: hypnosis was effective in reducing anxiety in six of seven studies dealing with both pain and anxiety.

Comparative treatment studies have revealed at least equi-valent if not better outcomes of hypnosis over alternate treatment procedures for anxiety in pediatric pain. For example, Kuttner (1988) found that a hypnotic trance involving a favorite story was more effective than either behavioral distraction or standard medical practice in alleviating pain and anxiety of bone marrow transplants in young children. This benefit was sustained on sub-sequent medical procedures. A randomized control study by Liossi & Hatira (1999) of 30 children undergoing bone marrow aspirations revealed that hypnosis was more effective than coping skills training as far as reducing anxiety, and both these interventions were more effective than no intervention in reducing pain and pain-related anxiety from baseline to treatment.   Wall & Womack (1989) trained 20 pediatric oncology patients to use self-directed hypnosis (without being told that it was hypnosis) or active cognitive strategy for pain and anxiety during medical procedures.   Both strategies reduced pain but neither reduced anxiety.

The effects of hypnosis are quite likely moderated by client variables such as suggestibility and age.   In an ethnically diverse sample of children with cancer or blood disorders, hypnotizable children showed significantly lower pain, anxiety, and distress in response to hypnosis than did low hypnotizable children (Smith et al. 1996).   Kuttner et al. (1988) randomly assigned 59 children from two age groups (3-6 and 7-20) to 3 conditions: hypnotic imaginative involvement, behavioral distraction, or standard medical practice.   Each intervention was repeated.   At the first point of intervention, the younger group given hypnosis showed significant reductions in distress/anxiety, whereas the older group in both treatment conditions showed significant reductions in pain and anxiety.   At the second intervention, both the groups showed reductions.

Among adults, the results have been no less supportive of hypnosis as an intervention on anxiety associated with pain. Hypnosis produced almost total relief of symptoms including anxiety and pain in 68% of 37 patients hospitalized for various medical diseases (Kaye & Schindler, 1990).   In a study of 51 cases referred for pain and symptom management (Sokel, Lansdown & Kent, 1990) 36 were taken on for training in self-hypnotherapy; of these, 29 were rated as improved or much improved after two to three sessions (Faymonville et al. (1997) randomly assigned 60 patients receiving elective plastic surgery under local anesthesia and intravenous sedation to a hypnosis or control condition.   Peri- and postoperative anxiety and pain were significantly lower in the hypnosis group which also reported an impression of enhanced intraoperative control as compared to control patients. Mairs (1995) found that primigravida women trained in hypnosis showed significantly lower ratings of pain and anxiety postbirth as compared to primigravida women who did not receive hypnosis training. Even cancer patients receiving hypnosis to ease pain and anxiety associated with bone marrow aspirations, lumbar punctures, and chemotherapeutic injections achieved significant reductions in multiple measures of pain and anxiety after hypnosis training (Kellerman, Zeltzer, Ellenberg & Dash, 1983).

As the cumulative evidence reveals, the beneficial effects of hypnotherapy on anxiety and pain seem to generalize across different types of painful conditions notwithstanding variations in the type of hypnosis. For example, Gabert and Uwe (1991) used Milton Erickson's interspersal hypnotic technique and Gordon's (1966) therapeutic metaphor on 56 male and female university students undergoing cold pressor pain. VanDyck et al. (1991) used future-oriented hypnotic imagery within a framework of autogenic suggestion to achieve significantly reduced state anxiety, depression, and pain medication usage in 55 tension headache patients (18-60 years old). After controlling for relaxation and imagery, hypnotizability scores correlated significantly with reductions in pain ratings. Yet further variations in hypnotherapy are available for implementation towards anxiety reduction in pain sufferers.

Systematic Desensitization. Systematic desensitization has been a treatment of choice for anxiety, especially phobias. It works by reciprocal inhibition, because relaxation diffuses anxiety as much as anxiety diminishes relaxation. Of course, the replacement of anxiety or tension with relaxation is a gradual progression in modest and attainable steps. The individual is systematically desensitized by relaxing in response to an image of the least feared stimulus, then a more-feared stimulus in the anxiety hierarchy, and so on until the most feared stimulus is tackled. This is particularly suited to the management of anxiety associated with pain, where imaginal exposure to the noxious stimulus is much more practical and innocuous than in vivo exposure to the same stimulus.

In the context of pain-related anxiety, only one study appears to have utilized systematic desensitization. Kondas & Scetnicka (1972) assigned two matched groups of pregnant women (with heightened anxiety about childbirth) to either a systematic desensitization condition or psychoprophylaxis. Anxiety declined in both groups, but more so in the desensitization group which further evidenced a significant reduction in pain intensity and duration of labor.

Stress Inoculation.   Stress Inoculation is a cognitive-behavioral approach developed by Meichenbaum and Turk (1976) that has applicability for various types of emotional distress as well as pain. It involves training in multiple skills such as reappraisal and relaxation across three phases: education, rehearsal, and application. Individuals prepare for the noxious event, practice coping self-statements and techniques such as relaxation, and then use them as needed during the actual event.

A few studies demonstrate the efficacy of this procedure in treating pain-related anxiety. The first is a case study of an 11-year-old girl who participated in stress inoculation training for dental anxiety (Nelson, 1981). Her actual "in chair" behavior and subjective reports of anxiety improved , these being maintained for up to five and a half months later. In a nomothetic study of 24 surgery patients, stress inoculation training reduced anxiety and pain and improved postoperative adjustment including reduced analgesic medication and recovery time (Wells, Howard, Nowlin & Vargas,1986). A more recent study by Ross & Berger (1996) showed that stress inoculation training led to significantly less postsurgical pain and anxiety in injured athletes undergoing arthroscopic surgery compared to a similar group receiving physical therapy only.

Integrated Treatments.   Just as stress inoculation combines multiple techniques for the alleviation of anxiety, other attempts at integrating techniques for anxiety reduction have emerged. Some of the resulting packages comprise techniques with already demonstrated worth and others incorporate new techniques.   The rules of combination may not always be clear but the outcome seems to be consistently good.

One example is a case study by Daniels (1976) in which autohypnosis was combined with covert modeling and covert re-inforcement to reduce dental anxiety in a 37-year-old female with postoperative pain.   In a larger sample of 23 chronic pain outpatients, Khatami & Rush (1982) implemented a treatment package of symptom control, stimulus control, and social system modification.   The 14 patients who completed the full course of therapy over an average of 23 weekly hour-long sessions achieved significant decreases in anxiety, depression, pain, and medication intake.

Several other studies have appeared in which anxiety was treated under the general rubric of cognitive-behavior therapy (CBT).   It is difficult to identify the specific ingredients that went into such therapy but in all likelihood cognitive precursors of anxiety were addressed by reappraisal and behavioral consequents of anxiety were addressed by relaxation techniques.

One CBT program for unexplained chest pain incorporated breathing and relaxation training, identification and alteration of beliefs about the pain, behavioral experiments and problem-solving for social situations (Van Peski-Oosterbaan et al. 1997).   The patients who completed this treatment and follow-up at 6 and 12 months showed significant reduction in anxiety, pain, and functional limitations.   Basler & Rehfisch (1990) described an outpatient CBT program for chronic pain patients in three primary care practices in which the main focus was promotion of self-control strategies.   Compared to no-treatment controls, these patients improved in anxiety, depression, and physical symptoms.   Whether delivered individually or in a group, CBT seems to exert enduring effects on anxiety, for example in persons with long-term work-related upper limb pain (Spence, 1989) where gains were maintained at 6-month follow-up while being clearly absent in wait-listed controls.

Further, comparative studies have shown that CBT approaches to anxiety outperform other types of psychological interventions. Getka & Glass (1992) prescribed a CBT package to dental anxiety patients and found that this was not only more effective than a wait-listed control but also better than a group receiving a gentle style of treatment from dentists. Moreover, the changes in anxiety and other symptoms were apparent across multimodal measures, and the gains were not lost at follow-up one year later. In another study, rheumatoid arthritis patients who had received conventional medical treatment were assigned to one of three conditions: (i) thermal biofeedback and group CBT, (ii) structured social support group therapy, or (iii) no adjunct treatment. Both treatment groups showed significant decreases in trait anxiety and depression from pre- to posttreatment but only CBT subjects decreased significantly in pain behavior and self-reported pain intensity. Finally, a 3-week CBT-based multidisciplinary treatment program was implemented by McCracken & Gross (1998) to achieve functional restoration in 79 chronic pain patients. Patients improved on all outcome measures including pain-related anxiety at admission and general daily activity. Moreover, the reductions in pain-related anxiety significantly predicted overall functioning.

Pharmaceutical Interventions

Most of the medications for anxiety in pain patients currently revolve around a large group of drugs called benzodiazepines. These reduce the activity of the reticular activating system and other areas of the brain by the actions of GABA, the brain's major inhibitory neurotransmitter. The result is a reduction in neural activity and awareness and some promotion of muscle relaxation. Benzodiazepines currently approved by the Food and Drug

Administration in the U.S. are chlordiazepoxide, diazepam, oxazepam, clorazepate, lorazepam, prazepam, alprazolam, and halazepam. They have been used extensively but their success is tempered by their tendency to reduce anxiety at doses also producing sedation (Carvey, 1998). They should hence be carefully selected on the basis of the particular type of anxiety disorder in question. Phobias, for example are not effectively managed by the continued use of these drugs. Acute anxiety such as panic attacks may respond to alprazolam, clonazepam, and lorazepam. For generalized anxiety, long-acting, low potency benzodiazepines (e.g., diazepam 15-30 mg/day) or even buspirone (a nonbenzodiazepine) are preferred (Maxmen, 1991).

Several applications of anxiolytic drugs in pain patients have been documented. A classic study is that by Chapman & Feather (1973) who found that diazepam significantly reduced the anxiety associated with intense tourniquet pain as contrasted to placebo but not when pitted against aspirin. Diazepam also had no effects on sensory sensitivity to radiant heat pain. The implication is that diazepam exerts its impact on the affective but not the sensory component of pain.

While the benzodiazepines are among the safest of anxiolytic drugs, the limits of their efficacy should be noted. They are best used for short periods of less than a week. Beyond that, efficacy is not likely to increase with dosage escalation. This tolerance to the drug is not merely psychological but also physiologic as verified by the reduced ability of the drug to enhance chloride conductance (Yu, Chiu, & Rosenberg, 1988). Along with the dependence on the drug, individuals at this stage are also likely to become more anxious about the failure of the drug to produce its initial effects. Sudden cessation or reduction of the drug can produce withdrawal in the form of subtle perceptual distortions, headache, and insomnia (Owen & Tyrer, 1983) which may develop over several weeks because of the long half-life of the drug. Addiction is a risk only if the drug is abused at high doses especially for recreational purposes (Griffiths & Sannerud, 1987). Dellemijn & Fields (1994) have also detected evidence of high doses of benzodiazepines causing depression in normals, although this is yet to be investigated in pain patients.

Apart from the limits to efficacy, the side effects of benzodiazepines cannot be ignored. As outlined in Maxmen (1991), the most common of these are light-headedness (in 6.8% to 30% of users), dry mouth and throat (12.6%), headache (9.1%) tachycardia (7.7%), palpitations (7.7%), nausea and vomiting (7.4%), constipation (7.1%) and diarrhea (7%). As with all sedative-hypnotic drugs, psychological functioning is affected. Cognitive processes such as judgment, concentration, insight, and planning are all blunted as the dosage increases (Carvey, 1998). Central nervous system effects on behavior include clumsiness in 20% of users and fatigue in 18% (Maxmen, 1991).

One class of drugs most widely used to treat pain that also exerts an ameliorative effect on anxiety are the opioids. In fact, Hill et al. (1952) reported that morphine reduced anxiety related to pain but under conditions without anxiety, morphine had little effect. A similar finding was reported by Kornetsky (1954) who found that morphine raised the differential threshold of pain when the subject was anxious but not otherwise. However, this old study used thermal pain and subjects with a history of opiate addiction.

There are extensive updates and reviews of the literature on anxiolytic medication. Most of these accounts are not specifically directed at the pain population, but they offer details about the mechanism, efficacy, and prescription guidelines for this class of drugs. The reader is referred to Sandford, Argyropoulos and Nutt (2000) and Bateson (2002) for basic pharmacology of anxiolytics. For applications to specific anxiety disorders, the reader might consider Blanco, Antia and Liebowitz (2002) and Westra and Stewart (2002).

Conclusion

Epidemiological data has accumulated to create a picture of anxiety as prevalent in about 60% of chronic pain sufferers but the statistics for acute pain sufferers are less forthcoming. More research needs to be done to address this issue of how anxiety prevalence rates vary as a function of the history of the pain, its etiology, and system of the body affected. Also important is the comparison of the pain population with other medical populations. Chances are that nearly all patients with physical or psychological disorders have anxiety -- perhaps clinically significant anxiety (if they're matched in terms of illness severity). So the question that arises is whether or not there is anything special about anxiety as a problem among those with pain.

Also important is the level of anxiety *relative to* other affective states such as anger, depression etc. Preliminary data is available on this (Fernandez, Clark, & Rudick-Davis, 1999; Fernandez & Milburn, 1994). In keeping with research on affective disorders, there appears to be comorbidity between anxiety and depression in pain patients too.

While research repeatedly suggests that where there is pain there is likely to be anxiety, what is more important at this stage is the particular nature of the interaction between anxiety and pain: is the anxiety a predisposing factor, a trigger, a correlate, an exacerbator, a consequence, or a perpetuating factor in pain? In this chapter, an attempt was made to organize the published research on anxiety and pain according to these categories. In some cases, the existing research does shed light on these questions, but in other cases, it is in its infancy and therefore ambiguous. Future research should be driven by á priori hypotheses about the specific interaction between anxiety and pain.

Another limitation of the body of research is the abundance of studies in which multiple measures have been intercorrelated out of which emerged a significant relationship between anxiety and pain. Incidental findings like these could be the result of familywise Type I error. Moreover, correlational research cannot bear on causality which is implied when one variable is a precursor or a consequence of another.

The measures of anxiety are a matter of much debate. Most studies in this area have relied on verbal report to the exclusion of other measures. Verbal report is indispensable in determining how a person feels but it is subject to distortion or even simulation. Behavioral observations and physiological measures, though not definitive, can help corroborate such verbal reports. According to Maddock, Carter, Tavano-Hall and Amsterdam (1998), even the adoption of a nosological system does not provide unequivocal grounds for a diagnosis of anxiety. They suspected that the diagnosis of panic disorder by psychiatric interview was debatable when 58% of a sample of normal coronary chest pain patients with negative scintigrams met DSM-III criteria for current panic disorder. This should not be taken to mean that physiological indices are better markers than verbal reports of anxiety or any other affective state for that matter. Neither is it sound to rely on one composite measure that may obscure important differences (DeGood, Buckelew & Tait, 1985). What is being proposed is that when multiple modalities of assessing anxiety converge they strengthen the confidence in a finding, and when they diverge they lead the researcher to alternative explanations or caveats. Along these lines, behavioral observations also add a great deal to the quantification of anxiety (LeBaron & Zelter, 1984).

There is also concern about the applicability of certain questionnaires for assessing anxiety in the pain population. The venerable State-Trait Anxiety Inventory has been widely used but its items do not relate to pain in particular. A new generation of anxiety-assessing instruments pertinent to pain has emerged. However, these may need further adaptation according to the specific pain population being studied. Zelter & LeBaron (1986), for example, argue that problems unique to children and adolescents undergoing treatment for catastrophic diseases call for unique assessment methods.

The mechanism by which anxiety causes or is caused by pain can be pieced together based on research from psychology as well as biology. Models of overattention and overprediction have been proposed as have explanations related to muscle activity and vascular factors. However, it would be interesting to explore the precise cognitive appraisals that underlie anxiety in pain sufferers. Appraisals about the cause of the patient's condition and its implications for functioning and life itself are intimately linked to the experience of pain. Yet, research has been scant in this area, thus limiting our abilities to understand and help patients reinterpret their pain.

By far, the treatment of anxiety in pain sufferers has attracted more research attention than just about any other issue in this area. A range of treatment techniques has emerged superior to control conditions. This raises the further possibility of combining these techniques to maximize efficacy. However, indiscriminate eclecticism is not advisable. Rather, techniques need to be carefully selected on the basis of their unique effects. This calls for more comparative research to gauge the differential efficacy of techniques. Additionally, techniques must be selected on the basis of theoretical and practical compatibility, and then meaningfully sequenced so that each technique builds on the other to produce a cumulative effect.

One subcategory of pain patients in special need of anxiety regulation is the panic-disordered chest pain sufferer. Specialized knowledge has accumulated from psychological research on panic that is yet to be applied to chest pain patients who do not have organic pathology. These individuals do not respond to cognitive restructuring alone or relaxation per sé or to imaginal desensitization (Marks, 1971). Instead, they require the addition of a strong dose of behavior modification through exposure therapy. Specifically, this takes the form of interoceptive exposure or the re-creation of physical sensations of panic within a clinical situation (Barlow, Craske, & Cerny, 1989). For example, the patient may be asked to walk a treadmill to produce cardiovascular sensations or s/he may be rotated in a swivel chair to produce audiovestibular sensations also associated with panic. Within the safety of the clinical situation, the patient realizes that there is no danger posed by these sensations. However, the reality-testing is only complete when the patient re-creates these sensations in naturalistic settings and ultimately becomes comfortable with experiencing them without anxiety or panic. Such in vivo exposure leads to habituation on the part of the patient. Barlow and Brown (1996) emphasize that this approach integrates the behavioral and the cognitive since patients are also trained to correct their overestimation of danger and various cognitive distortions about chest pain. Their review of the research shows a positive outcome in the vast majority of patients after 10 to 12 sessions of such panic control treatment. Moreover, this effect is maintained for up to two years of follow-up despite dramatic reductions in anxiolytic medication. This remains one of the best success stories in psychological treatments, and further application of these findings to the pain population would be appropriate.

Finally, there is a need to synthesize some of the literature in the field at a quantitative level, and meta-analysis presents an option here. Two areas that could benefit from meta-analysis are the research on (i) correlation between levels of anxiety and pain, and (ii) the efficacy of treatment techniques in alleviating anxiety of pain sufferers. In the case of the former, certain conflicting findings could be resolved, and in the case of the latter, a better idea of differential efficacy could be obtained.

CHAPTER 4

Depression and Pain

Definition and Conceptualization

At the core of depression are subjective feelings of sadness. Yet, depression is more than just sadness. It is viewed as a clinical syndrome in which the sadness is profound or sustained and combined with other biobehavioral symptoms. Cumulatively, these symptoms become maladaptive or impair the individual's day-to-day functioning.

For present purposes, the term depression is used in the same sense as the diagnostic label that goes by that name in psychiatric nosology. The nosological system used by most scholars and clincians in this area is the Diagnostic and Statistical Manual of Mental Disorders or DSM. The current version of this manual, DSM-IV-TR, (American Psychiatric Association, 2000) lists two main types of depression: major depression and dysthymia.

Major depression consists of at least two weeks of depressed mood (i.e. sadness, feelings of discouragement, hopelessness etc.) or loss of interest in most activities. In addition, there must be at least four of the following symptoms: weight loss, insomnia or hypersomnia, psychomotor retardation or agitation, fatigue, feelings of guilt, inadequacy or worthlessness, diminished concentration or ability to think, and recurrent thoughts of death. Major depression is also regarded as episodic: whether it occurs once or recurs, it is separated by at least two consecutive months when not all the criteria are met.

The second depressive disorder, dysthymia, refers to depressed mood for most of the time, most days and lasting at least two years. In addition, at least two of the following symptoms must be present: increased or decreased appetite, insomnia or hypersomnia, anergia or fatigue, low self-esteem, poor concentration or indecisiveness, and feelings of hopelessness. In other words, this is much like chronic, mild depression. Because of their habitually gloomy, brooding, bored presentation, individuals in this category are sometimes regarded as having a disturbance of temperament rather than an affective disorder (Akiskal, 1981, 1996).

Depressive manifestations may also occur as part of an adjustment disorder, in which case a diagnosis of adjustment disorder with depressed mood is given. This is characterized by sadness, tearfulness or feelings of hopelessness in response to an identifiable stressor occurring within three months of the onset of the stressor and resolving within six months of the termination of the stressor. The depressed mood and associated behaviors are in excess of what would be expected from exposure to the stressor, or there is marked impairment in social or occupational functioning.

DSM-IV-TR also proposes three depressive categories in need of further study: minor depressive disorder, recurrent brief depressive disorder, and depressive personality disorder. Minor depressive disorder is characterized by at least 2 weeks of depressed mood (sadness, feelings of discouragement, hopelessness etc.) or loss of interest in most activities but unlike major depression, at least two but no more than five of the symptoms of depression are present. It is speculated that this symptom pattern is common in primary care settings and among individuals with medical ailments. Recurrent brief depressive disorder, on the other hand, is identical to major depression in the number and severity of symptoms but does not meet the two-week criterion for major depression. Finally, depressive personality disorder is associated with a pattern of depressive cognitions, feelings, and behaviors e.g., cheerlessness, brooding on unhappy thoughts, pessimism, guilt, and low self-esteem. This begins by early adulthood and is not specific to any particular situation nor is it exclusive to a depressive episode as such.

Other nosological systems may not be structured exactly like the DSM but they share consensus on the main subtypes of depression. As some of these will be referred to in this chapter, they deserve mention here. The RDC (Research Diagnostic Criteria) propounded by Spitzer, Endicott and Robins (1978) uses the diagnoses of major depression, minor depression, intermittent depression, and endogenous/nonendogenous depression. These are defined a bit more stringently than in DSM. For example, RDC criteria for major depression require a few more symptoms and their presence for one week. The RDC category of intermittent depression is comparable to dysthymia in DSM. The RDC category called minor depression includes depressed mood and symptoms that do not reach the proportions of major depression but possess an episodic quality that contrasts with dysthymia. It is comparable to what is referred to in DSM as atypical depression.

Endogenous depression is supposedly biochemical in origin, whereas nonendogenous or reactive depression is more akin to neuroses. The latter, according to Charatan (1975) tends to emerge from some kind of loss, whether real or imagined. Similar terms have been used by psychoanalysts but with different meanings. For example, Schmale (1972) distinguishes between endogenous depression (depressive symptoms resulting from a turning in of aggression onto the self) and exogenous depression (depressive symptoms that prevent a reawakening of pain from infantile separation).

Building on psychoanalytic foundations, Arieti (1962) emphasized that "depression is the reaction to loss of what we consider a normal ingredient of our psychologic life" (p. 397) so that what is lost could be a loved person, the love of this person, a symbolic situation, a status, self-concept, or an ideal. However, the reaction can be of two different kinds: an aggressively dependent kind of depression called "claiming depression", or a self-accusative kind called "self-blaming depression" (Arieti, 1962). The former is ultimately a plea by the depressed for help from the dominant other; this takes the form of gigantic demands such as "Don't abandon me", "You have the means to help me",

"If I suffer, it is because you do not relieve my suffering". Any unfulfilled claim is experienced as a wound or loss that brings about depression. The self-blaming depression, on the other hand occurs more often in those with a sense of duty, sin, guilt, and punishment. Theirs is not so much a plea for help as an expression of atonement as in "I do not need help or your pity", and "I deserve to die". The self-blame is part of a need for atonement as a means of achieving self-redemption. This distinction between "claiming" versus "self-blaming" depression is parallel to the present-day distinction between extra-punitive versus intra-punitive anger. Depression, like anger, can be other-directed or self-directed in its action tendency.

Iovchuk (1985-86) found that in childhood depression, the clinical picture was complicated by a greater variability in symptoms and their susceptibility to external influences. Due to the fragmentary nature of the depressive symptoms in children, six types of depression were identified: somaticized depression, anxious-agitated depression, depression with fear, dysphoric depression, depressive pseudofeeblemindedness, and sluggish-adynamic depression.

Covino et al. (1983) claims as many as 13 distinct patterns of depression in pain sufferers, asthmatics, and tuberculosis patients. This is based on an O-type cluster analysis of subscales of the MMPI Scale 2 developed at the Massachusetts Mental Health Center.

There are also subtypes based on subsets of depressive symptoms. Relying on clinical observations, von Brauchitsch (1975) has identified a depressive state in which mental symptoms predominate without concomitant alterations in mood. These symptoms include impaired concentration, and disinterest in life or its activities, plus disturbance in sleep, libido, and appetite. It is highly debatable whether this qualifies as a mental rather than affective disturbance, but von Brauchitsch characterizes this condition as fundamentally a problem of volition. Others too have made a case for this as a subtype of depression, giving it labels such as "pseudo-anergic syndrome" (Karno & Hoffman, 1974).

Not dissimilar is what Chaturvedi (1989) refers to as "psychalgic depressive disorder" as observed in pain patients. Here, the predominant depressive symptoms are disinterest in surroundings, early morning awakenings, reduced appetite, and even suicidal ideation.

The emerging picture here is that depression as operationalized by DSM embodies a host of symptoms, not all of which are always present in any single individual. Subgroups of symptoms can be identified; these may not be purely cognitive since cognition influences affect, which in turn has motivational, behavioral, and physiological concomitants. The divisions may be along other boundaries (e.g., "agitated" versus "retarded" depressives), which justify the specification of subtypes of depression. Such a reconceptualization may help reduce the sometimes conflicting or confusing findings relating depression to pain and other disorders.

Depressive Features

The prevailing view is that mood disturbance is the defining feature of depression (Widlocher, 1983). This refers to subjective feelings of sadness as well as degrees of helplessness and hopelessness. However, Widlocher (1983) has also suggested that psychomotor retardation might be the major response in depressive conditions. This is similar to what Schmale (1972) terms the "conservation-withdrawal" reaction to depression. It includes the general slowing down of motor movements, speech and mental functions. Such slowing down of activity need not be an epiphenomenon of dysphoric mood.

Observing about a dozen 24-65 year-old depressed inpatients and examining data from an additional 50 depressed patients, Silber, Rey, Savard & Post (1980) noted changes in the form of language and thinking that reflected serious disturbances in ego functioning. Specifically, patients evidenced a restricted ability to express or experience a range of affect. The authors suggested that such affective inaccessibility might be the prime feature of severe and/or prolonged depression.

Depression as an Associated/Defining Feature of Chronic Pain

Along with alcoholics, advanced cancer patients, and those with a history of affective disorder, pain patients are among the populations at highest risk of depression (Massie & Holland, 1990). This contrasts with pain-free individuals who are far less likely to report depression (Hodgkiss, Watson & Sufraz, 1994; Naidoo & Pillay, 1994). A contrast can also be made between acute pain which tends to be associated with anxiety (Meilman, 1984) versus chronic pain which is largely associated with depression (Lipowski, 1990a), in particular, reactive depression (Sternbach, 1975). Most change in depression occurs within the first three months of pain onset (Philips & Grant, 1991) and can settle down thereafter, but when the pain lasts 25 years or more ("ancient pain" as it is called), patients are even more likely to be diagnosed with depression as compared to the average chronic pain sufferer (Swanson, Maruta & Wolff, 1986). Depression is often regarded by chronic pain patients themselves as one of their worst problems, in some cases, leading them to contemplate suicide (Hitchcock, Ferrell & McCaffery, 1994).

Epidemiology

As mentioned in Chapter 1, epidemiology is the study of the distribution of a disease, its natural history, and co-factors of the disease in a population. Thus, it encompasses statistics about the prevalence, incidence, and mortality rate of a disease in a specified group, its course over time, and its relationship to demographics (such as gender and age) and to behavior.

The Course of Depression in Pain Sufferers

As explained in the previous chapter, pain at the time of its onset triggers much anxiety. This gives way to frustration and anger as the pain recurs or becomes prolonged (as explained in the next chapter). However, when pain becomes chronic or terminal, it is more likely to be associated with depression. Hendler (1984) has asserted that depression is absent in the acute stage of pain less than two months in duration. It is also relatively rare in the subacute stage between two and six months when hypochondriasis and hysteria predominate. Rather, it is the chronic stage of pain (6 months to 8 years) when depression takes hold, finally giving way to resignation and a diminution of depressive symptoms as the pain persists even further. This sequence may parallel the cognitive changes in self-esteem and helplessness as the pain goes from acute to chronic (Skevington, 1993). Turner and Romano (1984) posit that depression tends to have a rapid onset in chronic pain patients, dissipating slowly over 3-5 years.

Prevalence of Depression in Pain

Apart from the natural history described above, it helps to know what percentage of those in pain have depression. Most reviewers of the pain-depression literature state that there is high comorbidity between these two conditions but go on to point out the high variability in epidemiological statistics of co-occurring pain and depression. By some accounts, the prevalence of depression in the pain population ranges from 30% to 87% (Smith, 1992), by others it ranges from 10% to 100% (Romano & Turner, 1985). In fact, the range is even wider from as low as 0% (Ehlert, Heim & Hellhammer, 1999) to the very peak of 100% (Violon, 1980). This incredible variability may be due to sampling error arising from heterogeneous groups of pain patients and methodological differences in data collection. Such inconsistent findings shed little light on the relationship between pain and depression. Clearly, it is not enough to extract statistics from studies without at least relating them to the peculiarities of the sample in question. By separating the epidemiological statistics according to types of pain, greater internal consistency of results might emerge. Therefore, an attempt is made here to bring some order to the epidemiological data by organizing the relevant studies into subgroups distinguished primarily by the type of patients sampled. The common denominator across pain patients in these studies is that all had some form of chronic pain, but beyond that they differed in important ways as detailed later. Unless otherwise stated, the rates of depression reported here are point prevalence estimates. Where possible, these are pitted against prevalence statistics for control or comparison groups.

Depression in the Community

Any evaluation of the prevalence of depression in a sample must be done with reference to a benchmark. To this end, it is instructive to consider the depression statistics in the general community. According to the American Psychiatric Association (2000), the point prevalence of major depression in community samples of adults is about 2% to 3% for men and between 5% and 9% for women; for dysthymia, the prevalence is about 3%. By comparison, the prevalence of depressive disorders is higher in medical populations especially the chronic pain population.

Depression in Medical Populations

How can epidemiological data more convincingly show that it is the pain of chronic pain patients that is responsible for the relatively high rates of depression found in this group? One way is to pit the depression rates in pain patients against those of a meaningful comparison group -- a group with no pain that is otherwise similar. Appropriate comparison groups may be located in the general medical population.

In a primary care population, the rates of depressive disorders tend to be relatively low. Of 1072 patients seen in primary care facilities, 5.8% had major depression, 3.4% had minor depression, and 5% had intermittent depression, as defined by RDC and DSM-III criteria (Hoeper, Nyczi, Cleary, Regier and Goldberg, 1979). In a smaller sample of 294 primary care patients, 9.2% had some depressive disorder as defined by DSM-III (Schulberg, Saul, McClelland, Ganguli, Christy & Frank, 1985). Wells, Golding and Burnham (1988) surveyed 11,000 patients seen by doctors in solo practices or in health maintenance organizations, and found approximately 2500 to have depressive symptoms, 312 of these meeting criteria for a mood disorder; in other words, only about 3% had diagnosable depression.

Among general medical inpatients, the rates of depression are higher. The intermediate cutoff for depression on the CES-D (Center for Epidemiological Study-Depression Scale; Radloff, 1977) was attained by 35% of general medical patients (Fava et al. 1982). A comparable cutoff for the Beck Depression Inventory (Beck et al., 1961) was attained by 32% (Cavanaugh, 1983), and 38% of general medical patients (Rosenberg et al. 1988).

For specific diseases, rates of depression are consistently high among poststroke victims. In one study of such patients (Robinson & Price, 1982), 29% attained the cutoff score for depression on the General Health Questionnaire-28; in another similar sample (Sinyor, Amato, Kaloupek, Becker, Goldenberg, & Coopersmith, 1986), 22% attained a high score of at least 60 on the Zung (Zung, 1965); in a third sample (Wade, Leigh-Smith & Hewer, 1987), 20% attained a high cutoff of 19 on the Wakefield Self-Assessment Depression Inventory (Snaith, Ahmed, Melita & Hamilton, 1971). In endstage renal disease, intermediate-to-high scores of depression were attained by 26% of patients given the BDI (Rodin & Voshart, 1987) and 27% given the Zung (Kutner, Fair & Kutner, 1985). Other conditions such as Parkinson's Disease and gynecological ailments were associated with variable rates of depression.

The pattern of increase in prevalence of major depression from community to primary care to inpatient medical populations has been traced by Katon & Sullivan (1990). Their data reveal an estimated 4.8% to 9.2% of ambulatory primary care patients as having major depression. Between 20% and 45% of cancer patients had major depression and/or generalized anxiety disorder. For those with stroke, the prevalence of major/minor depression is about 25% climbing to about 30% at six months follow-up. In the case of myocardial infarction, about 45% had major/minor depression shortly after admission to hospital, this figure dropping to 33% three-to-four months later.

Pain Patients Versus Medical Populations

Is depression greater in pain patients than in other medical populations? Of the studies making *direct* comparisons of pain and pain-free patients, a few have found differences in the predicted direction (e.g., Spear, 1967) but more have found trends in the opposite direction (e.g., Pilling, et al. 1967; Pelz, Merskey, Brant & Haselting, 1981). However, as pointed out by Romano and Turner (1985), it is probably difficult to make a decision on these grounds because many of the studies did not match groups on important attributes such as age, socioeconomic status, etc. It is also naïve to assume that just because some patients do not have pain they naturally suffer less from depression. Every disease has its own morbidity. There may be many other symptoms (some even more troublesome than pain) that may be responsible for depression. These range from physical difficulties like fatigue, disfigurement, insomnia, and sexual dysfunction, to psychosocial adversities such as isolation and ostracism, the financial burden of medical costs, occupational disruption, and an overall decline in self-esteem. Any one of these taken to an extreme can produce equivalent or greater depression compared to that produced by pain alone. Then, there are multiple problems unrelated to the patient's illness but no less responsible for depression. Interpersonal difficulties with the family, on the job, and in social contexts can tangentially enter into the picture compounding the depression.

As in other medical ailments, the rates of depression in pain patients are expected to climb from community samples to primary care to specialty clinics. In chronic low back pain patients for example, depression prevalence is as low as 26% for those seen in general practice (Love, 1987) and as high as 78% for those in specialty pain clinics (Sullivan & D'Eon, 1990).

Non-referred pain sufferers. Extrapolating from the above pattern, depression rates may be expected to vary with the referral status of the pain patients. Research shows that these rates are lowest in those not yet referred for treatment. Magni (1984) found that of 64 factory workers with chronic low back pain, 11% had current major depression. Drawing from a pool of 1016 people enrolled in a health maintenance organization, Dworkin et al. (1990) found a 1% prevalence of major depression in those with only one chronic pain complaint. This figure rose to 9% for those with two chronic pain complaints, and 12% for those with three chronic pain complaints.

Patients referred to pain clinics. Compared to pain patients in primary care, those referred to pain clinics generally have a greater prevalence of depression. Of 20 patients referred to a multidisciplinary pain consultation service, 50% had major depression (Schaffer, 1980) and of 40 chronic pain patients referred to a pain center, 30% met criteria for major depressive episode (Turner & Romano, 1984). A larger sample of 172 patients attending the Auckland Pain Clinic in New Zealand witnessed a similar 30% prevalence of depression (Large, 1980).

The prevalence rates seem to be even higher in studies of larger samples. Lindsay & Wyckoff (1981) reported that of 300 patients referred to a pain program, 87% were diagnosable with some form of depression. In another sample of 182 chronic pain patients referred to a pain program, 56% had some type/s of depressive disorder (Fishbain et al. 1986). So, there is consensus that depression rates are higher in the pain population than in the general population. However, the type of depression in these patients is not clear.

Using the RDC to differentiate subtypes of depression, Davidson, Krishnan, France & Pelton (1985) performed a controlled study of 57 chronic pain sufferers (mostly inpatients with back pain). Results showed that 42% had major depression, 37% had minor or intermittent depression, and the remaining 21% had no depression. Only in 12% of the pain patients with major depression, or 5% of the total sample, was the depression endogenous, and that too by liberal RDC criteria.

Consecutive referrals to pain clinics. Instead of randomly selecting patients from a pain clinic at one point in time, some investigators have studied a string or succession of patients referred to pain clinics over a period of time. For example, Kramlinger, Swanson & Maruta (1983) studied 100 patients referred consecutively to a hospital-based pain program. Of these, 25 satisfied criteria for major depression as defined by Research Diagnostic Criteria (RDC), 39 were regarded as probably depressed, and the rest were deemed not depressed. The same criteria employed in another 100 consecutive referrals to the same inpatient pain program, revealed 34 as definitely depressed, 20 as probably depressed, and the rest not depressed (Maruta, Vatterott & McHardy, 1989). Haley, Turner & Romano (1985) found that of 63 patients at a pain clinic, 49% had major depression. This is similar to findings by Rudy, Kerns and Turk (1988) that 50% of a sample of 100 consecutive referrals to a pain clinic evidenced at least moderate levels of depression. In an outpatient sample of 126 chronic pain patients consecutively appearing at three pain clinics, 68% scored high enough on the CES-D to warrant a diagnosis of major depression (Arnstein, Caudill, Mandle, Norris & Beasley, 1999).

Psychiatric referrals. Some pain patients are specifically referred to a psychologist or psychiatrist. It is to be expected that this subgroup would have even higher rates of depression than those referred to a pain clinic. In a New Zealand study by Large (1986), chronic pain patients scoring high on affective disturbance or illness affirmation as measured by the Illness Behavior Questionnaire (Pilowsky & Spence, 1983) were referred for psychiatric interview. The sample consisted of 15 men and 35 women with a modal age of 45-54 years old and a mean pain chronicity of about 5 years. They underwent a semi-structured interview of about 90 minutes to 2 hours, at the conclusion of which a DSM-III diagnosis was delivered. The inter-judge reliability of the clinical diagnosis was high on Axis I but moderate for Axis II.

More Depressed Than the Depressed?

We now know that compared to the general community, chronic pain sufferers have higher rates of depression, especially if they are patients seen at a pain clinic. A further question that arises is "How does the depression of pain patients compare with that of depressed patients in general?" This is the subject matter for a controlled study. In a small-scale comparison of 13 patients with chronic pain and depression versus an equal number of matched controls with depression but no pain, the former turned out significantly more depressed than the control group (Mohamad, Weisz, & Waring, 1978). However, Davidson et al. (1985) found that compared to a similar-aged control group of 35 depressed inpatients without pain, 57 chronic pain patients had significantly less frequent vegetative symptoms of depression, including sleep disturbance, libido change, diurnal variation, and appetite change. In pain patients who did have major depression, the neurovegetative symptoms (as measured by scores on the Hamilton Depression Inventory) were comparable to those in their pain-free depressed counterparts.   So, while prevalence of depression is greater in pain patients, morbidity is not necessarily so.

Depression by Pain Type

Head pain. Of the different types of pain, one that stands out as most associated with depression is head pain. Violon (1980) found depression in 84% of subjects with headaches and 100% of those with atypical facial pain. This is consistent with the results of Diamond's (1964) survey revealing 84% of headache sufferers to have depressive symptoms. A similar pattern has been noted by Cox and Thomas (1981), and in recent reports of correlations between head pain and depression (Faravelli, Masini & Poli, 1979; Ziegler, Rhodes & Hassanein, 1978). According to Sagduyu and Sahiner (1997), the rates of depression may be particularly high when the migraine and tension-type headache occur chronically in the absence of organic pathology.

Back pain. Krishnan et al. (1985) used RDC criteria to assess types of depression in 71 chronic low back pain patients. Of these, 31 were diagnosed with major depression, 8 with minor depression, and 18 with intermittent depressive disorder. Love (1987) found that in a sample of 68 chronic low back pain patients, 25% reported major depression. Engel, Von Korff & Katon (1996) surveyed 1059 enrolees in a health maintenance organization (HMO) who consecutively presented at one of the participating clinics with back pain (including pain of thoracic and cervical spine). A telephone administration of the depression subscale of the Symptom Checklist-90, Revised (SCL-90-R; Derogatis, 1977) revealed that about 63% of the sample scored less than 1.0 on the depression subscale, about 20% scored 1.01-1.6, and about 17% exceeded a score of 1.6. It is unclear what this means in relation to the maximum score of 5, but the authors offered the interpretation that "Lower levels of depressive symptoms were typical, but an appreciable proportion of patients reported moderate to severe depressive symptoms" (1996, p.199).

Maruta, et al. (1976) found that 38% of low back pain patients were depressed. A more recent controlled study of men with low back pain found a 22% prevalence of depression over a six-month period, and a 32% lifetime prevalence of depression.

Miscellaneous pain syndromes. To incorporate the less common varieties of pain and pain affecting multiple sites, a separate category can be formed. This miscellaneous group is associated with even greater variability in prevalence of depression. Of 36 patients with pain in head and neck, trunk or extremities, 28 were clinically depressed (Wilson, Blazer & Nashold, 1976). Of 34 patients with painful shoulder syndrome, 76% had clinically significant depression (Tyber, 1974). In a sample of patients with irritable bowel syndrome, 31% had depression but it is unclear if all these patients were in pain (Latimer, 1983). Monti et al. (1998) found that when controlling for the age of patients, complex regional pain syndrome and low back pain were both similar in terms of pain intensity and duration as well as in depressive disorder.

Depression has often been suspected in those with pain in an amputated part of the body. Such phantom pain can be extremely difficult to treat but also compounded when it becomes a reminder of the lost body part. It is estimated that between 20 and 60% of phantom pain patients seen in surgery or rehabilitation clinics are clinically depressed (Kashani, Frank, Kashani, Wonderlich & Reid, 1983; Randall, Ewalt & Blair, 1945; Shukla, Sahu, Tripathi & Gupta, 1982). This is consistent with the later finding by Sherman, Sherman and Bruno (1987) that 10 out of 21 phantom pain patients had clinical levels of depression. Ehlert, Heim & Hellhammer (1999) reported no clinical depression in any of 26 patients with chronic pelvic pain, even though there was a high prevalence of sexual abuse. Delaplaine, Ifabumuyi, Merskey & Zarfas (1978) found that in 227 psychiatric hospital admissions, 86 had pain, and of these, 15 had endogenous or neurotic depression. In other words, 17% of these psychiatric pain patients were depressed.

Acute versus chronic pain. There is little disagreement with the idea that acute pain and chronic pain possess quite different affective qualities.   Anxiety tends to be the primary affective disturbance in the former while depression tends to predominate in the latter. As explained by Meilman (1984), this may be attributable to the greater degree of disability associated with chronic than acute pain.

Investigating Chinese low back pain patients, Lee et al. (1992) compared profiles of the MMPI (Hathaway & McKinley, 1943) from 15 patients with acute pain versus 15 patients with chronic pain.   While both groups had higher elevations than healthy controls on the neurotic triad of the MMPI, the chronic pain patients were clearly more depressed than their acute counterparts.

Organic versus functional pain. The evidence here is mixed, probably because the very foundations for an organic-functional distinction are weak. This dichotomy did not make a difference to depression rates for pain patients in general (Sternbach, Wolf, Murphy & Akeson, 1973) low back pain patients (McCreary, Turner & Dawson, 1977) or facial pain patients (Marbach & Lund, 1981).   However, in studies by Hanvik (1951) and Calsyn and Louks (1976), depression was more marked in the functional than the organic group of pain patients. Sagduyu & Sahiner (1997) found depressive disorders to be two to three times greater in headache and migraine sufferers without organic pathology as compared to those with organic pathology. Reesor & Craig (1988) too observed that patients with medically incongruent low back pain evidenced higher pain intensity and depression than patients with low back pain that was medically explainable, but these differences vanished when physical impairment and disability were controlled for. This indicates that whether the pain is functional or organic is less important than the degree of impairment -- in predicting the depression of chronic pain sufferers.

Depressives With Pain

While the preceding studies uncover the prevalence of depression in pain patients, the converse, pain in depressives, is also of interest. If pain is as common in depressed patients as depression is in pain patients, then, there is an even stronger case for the comorbidity of the two conditions. Spear (1967) reported that 56% of depressives admitted to a psychiatric clinic presented with pain as one of their symptoms. Singh (1968) uncovered evidence for some sort of pain in 65% of patients with depression as a major presenting problem. Ward, Bloom & Friedel (1979) found all of 16 depressed subjects to have chronic pain complaints; however, this sample is far too small for any epidemiological interpretations. The Lindsay & Wyckoff (1981) study found that 59% of 191 depressed patients had pain in the three months preceding diagnosis. A more extensive survey of 11,000 medical patients found that 35% of those with depressive symptoms also reported pain (Wells et al.1989). Von Knorring, Perris, Eisemann, Eriksson and Perris (1983) reported that of 140 patients hospitalized for depressive disorder, 46% had pain but in most of these cases, the pain was slight. The pain was only moderate in 66% of 51 geriatric patients with major depression (Magni, Schifano & Deleo, 1985); in contrast, only 34% of medical patients had moderate pain.

Gender Differences In Depression Among Pain Patients

It is well known that in the general population, depression is twice as commonly manifested in women as in men. The question of particular interest to us here is whether this gender difference in depression carries over into the chronic pain population as well. Several studies have looked into this possibility.

Davidson et al. (1985) found that in a group of about 50 chronic back pain patients, the prevalence of depression was twice as high in men as compared to women, except in those pain patients with minor or intermittent depression, where women outnumbered men by a multiple of 3. In a study by Kramlinger, Swanson & Maruta (1983), the group of depressed chronic pain patients had 18 women and 7 men, whereas the group of nondepressed chronic pain patients had 18 women and 18 men. Most other studies too (Keefe, Wilkins, Cook, Crisson et al. 1986; Magni, Moreschi, Rigatti-Luchini & Merskey, 1994; Von Knorring, Perris, Eismann, Eriksson, 1989) showed higher prevalence rates for female than male chronic pain patients.

Specific prevalence data for different types of depression by gender of pain patients has been obtained by Fishbain et al. (1986). They reported psychiatric diagnoses of 283 chronic pain patients consecutively admitted to the Comprehensive Pain Center of the University of Miami. During a three-day period of evaluation by multidisciplinary staff, patients underwent a two-hour semistructured psychiatric interview by a senior psychiatrist in order to determine DSM-III diagnoses. The results pertaining to gender differences in depressive disorders are shown in Table 2 which is adapted from Fishbain et al. (1986).

Table 2

Prevalence of Depressive Disorders in Pain Patients (based on Fishbain et al. 1986)

	Males (N=156) %	Females (N=127) %	Total (N=283) %
Diagnosis			
Major depression and bipolar disorder in remission	.6	2.4	1.5
Current major depression (single and recurrent)	3.8	5.5	4.6
Dysthymic Disorder	20.5	26.8	23.3
Current major depression (single and recurrent) plus cyclothymic disorder plus dysthymic disorder	25.0	33.4	28.2
Adjustment disorder with depressed mood	25.6	31.5	28.3
Total number of patients with current depression (major depression, dysthymic disorder, cyclothymic disorder, adjustment disorder with depressed mood	49.9 *	63.8 *	56.2

* statistically significant difference, p< .05

As can be seen, the pure depressive disorders (major depression and dysthymia) were found in about 25% of males and 32% of females. Why is it that the prevalence of depression is greater in female than male chronic pain patients? One possibility is that the overall prevalence of depression in women is higher than in men, and this simply carries over into any subset of the general population, be they pain patients, school teachers, or consumers at large.   Another possibility is that certain pain syndromes are unique to women, and these may be more depressiogenic than other pain syndromes.   For example, depression is more common in female-specific conditions such as chronic pelvic pain (Nolan, Metheny & Smith, 1992) and dyspareunia (Meana et al. 1998) than in the general female population.   This suggests that chronic or recurrent pain contributes to the relatively high probability of depression in women.   In other painful conditions too such as migraine, fibromyalgia, and temporomandibular disorders (TMD), women predominate and (at least in TMD) depression rates are higher than those for men with the same disorder (Vimpari, Knuutila, Sakki & Kivela, 1995).   The higher rates may also be related to the greater number of pains reported by women (Dworkin, Von Korff & LeResche, 1990) and the severity of pain as perceived by women -- compared to men whose depression tends to be fueled more by functional impairment than by pain report (Haley, Turner & Romano, 1985).   In any case, this indicates that comorbid pain and depression are more pervasive in women than men.

Age Differences in Depression Among Pain Patients

With age comes an increased likelihood of medical problems, some of these becoming chronic and thereby producing persistent pain, thus further increasing the risk of depression.   For example, osteoarthritis, rheumatism, and angina are more common as people age and pain is a predominant symptom in these conditions.   It has been estimated that 70-80% of older people have at least one chronic health problem that could be associated with pain (Sorkin, Rudy, Hanlon, Turk, & Steig, 1990; Thomas & Roy, 1999).   Estimates reveal a steady increase in pain with age from 25% of those aged 61-70, 29% of those aged 71-80, to 40% of those over 80 (Crook, Rideout and Brown, 1984).   An age-gender interaction has also been reported (Avery, Novy, Nelson & Berry, 1996), depression being more common in younger women and older men with chronic pain.

With the increased pain and disability of old age comes an increased risk of depression. In a study of the institutionalized aged, the amount of pain increased from those with no depression to those with minor depression and to those with major depression (Parmelee, Katz and Lawton, 1991). In a retrospective study of those in their last year of life (70% of whom were older than 65), Cartwright, Hockey and Anderson (1973) found that 66% had reported pain in their last year. Interviews of survivors of 200 deceased community residents (all over age 65) revealed an increase in pain from 37% at one year before death to 66% at one month before death (Moss, Lawton & Glicksman, 1991).

Yet, the increased susceptibility of the elderly to pain-associated depression is often overlooked. As Melding (1995) explains, this may be due to the myth that physical symptoms in the elderly are the product of somatization. If anything, some data suggest that the elderly are inclined to ignore mild chronic symptoms and reattribute them to a normal ageing process (Leventhal & Prochaska, 1986; Lipowski, 1990b).

The argument that emerges in explaining gender and age effects is as follows. The more pain there is (in terms of number of sites affected, chronicity, nonorganicity, and disability), the more depression there is. Females and older people tend to have multiple pains that are more persistent, disabling, and functional in nature. These subgroups are hence likely to show greater depression than their counterparts.

Cultural Variables in Depression Among Pain Patients

Comparisons among ethnic groups of pain patients with regard to depression have been scant. One study (Averill, Novy, Nelson & Berry, 1996) reported no differences between "white" versus "nonwhite" patients. Of course, this leaves much room for further differentiation of ethnicity. In a study of depressed Canadian subjects, the prevalence of pain was less in Canadian Indian and Inuit individuals than in Caucasians (Pelz, Merskey, Brant & Haselting, 1981).

Chaturvedi and Michael (1986) have reported on depression and pain in India. In a large sample of 500 consecutive patients attending a psychiatric clinic, they found that 18.6% had chronic pain as a predominant complaint and 45% presented with depressive neurosis. However, the exact intersection between these two subgroups is unclear. In comparison to the study of psychiatric pain by Delaplaine et al. (1978), pain was less common in psychiatric patients but depression was more common among these psychiatric pain patients.

Lee et al. (1992) found that in a sample of Chinese patients with low back pain, the usual chronic-acute determinants of depression were upheld, but the gender effect was not. In their study, male MMPI profiles reflected more depression than those of females. While this is not an epidemiological study per sé, it may suggest that depression is more intense (though not necessarily more pervasive) in men -- at least within a Chinese population. However, a larger scale study needs to be undertaken to test this hypothesis.

Epidemiological Conclusions and Issues for Further Research

Epidemiology is not only about compiling statistics but also about looking for patterns that might illuminate hidden relationships among variables. As for the relationship between pain and depression, a picture emerges if one closely examines the following data: the percentage of those in pain who have depression, comparing this to healthy controls and other medical patients who do not have pain, the percentage of those with depression who have pain, the number of other symptoms characterizing depression, and the number of other symptoms characterizing pain. This emergent picture is as follows:

1. Not all chronic pain patients are depressed, and depression is only one of many features of chronic pain.
2. Not all depressed people are in pain
3. Pain is only one of many features of depressed individuals
4. Yet, chronic pain is often followed by depression
5. Depression is sometimes characterized by pain (chronic, intermittent, or acute)
6. Therefore, it is more likely that (persistent) pain drives depression than vice versa.

Significance

The sensation of pain is a focal concern of the pain patient and his/her caregiver. Depression makes for an additional burden on the patient with chronic pain. Furthermore, it can exert a compounding effect on the perception of pain. It is also one of the more serious affective disorders in view of its impairment of function and its potential for self-destructiveness.

A seminal paper by Schonfeld, Verboncoeur, Fifer, Lipschutz, Lubeck & Buesching (1997) documents the effects of depression and other affective disorders on health and functioning. More than 6000 enrolees in a health maintenance organization completed a 52-item subset of anxiety and depression items from the SCL-90-R (Derogatis, 1983), and completed the SF-36 (Ware, Snow, Kosinski & Gandek, 1993) to assess eight areas of health-related functioning. In addition, participants were interviewed and their medical records consulted for diagnostic information. Consistent with other epidemiological findings, major depression occurred most frequently, both as a single disorder and as one of multiple disorders. It also had the most pronounced impact on scores of functioning, these being about 25 points below predicted scores for a reference group with no disorders. The health burden of depression was evident in the role-emotional scale of the SF-36 which pertains to emotional abilities in performing daily responsibilities and the role-physical scale which measures physical abilities to perform daily responsibilities. Even more striking was the finding that the health burden of depression was comparable to that of certain medical conditions. For example, low back pain has been shown to reduce physical functioning by 9.1 points on the SF-36 as compared to the reduction of 9.4 points for depression (Wells, Stewart, Hays, Burnam, Rogers, Daniels, Berry, Greenfield & Ware, 1989).

Health Care Utilization

In a prospective study, Katon et al. (1986) screened 147 primary care patients and then observed them within a year later. It was found that those with moderate to severe depression had significantly more hospital visits, more phone calls to the clinic, and more medical evaluations than the nondepressed control group.

In a subsequent study, Katon, Von Korff, Lin, Bush, & Ormel (1990) screened 1000 patients who were in the top 10% in terms of frequency of visits to primary care physicians. They observed an over-representation of depressed individuals in this group -- more than two thirds had major depression.

A more recent prospective study by Engel, Von Korff and Katon (1996) surveyed just over 1000 enrolees in a health maintenance organization (HMO) who consecutively presented with back or neck pain. Three-to-six weeks later, these patients were interviewed by telephone regarding various pain and psychosocial variables. It was found that depression assessed by a subscale of the Symptom Checklist-90 (SCL-90; Derogatis, 1977) significantly predicted the total costs of health care services received by these patients over the next 12 months. These costs were for all inpatient and outpatient pharmacy and radiology services including charges reimbursed by the HMO for services provided outside the system. It is unclear if this included psychotherapy for depression which may have even further augmented the relationship between depression and health care costs. Nevertheless, as the authors concluded, the findings of such research point to the significance of depression as a target for assessment and intervention in pain patients.

Functional Impairment

Aneshensel, Frerichs and Huba (1984) found that patients with high scores on a depression rating scale also perceived themselves as more physical ill. This is consistent with the reports of greater physical limitations among psychiatric patients than patients without psychiatric complaint, notwithstanding chronic medical conditions (Wells, Golding & Burnham, 1988). Craig and Van Natta (1983) reported a strong positive correlation between self-rated depression and number of disability days too. The combination of affective disturbance with somatic ailment seems to exert an even greater (additive) effect on perceived ill health, functional impairment, and social and vocational difficulties. Weickgenant, Slater, Patterson, Atkinson, Grant, and Garfin (1993) found that depressed chronic pain patients tended to avoid activities more than their nondepressed counterparts did; this in turn may hinder physical therapy and rehabilitation for chronic pain sufferers.

Mortality

Not only does depression carry a load of morbidity, it also increases mortality. Bruce and Leaf's (1989) study of a community sample of 3007 individuals (aged 50 or more) revealed more than four times the number of deaths in patients with major depression as compared to those without depression. This was over a 15-month follow-up period. A similar finding was reported in a prospective study of elderly patients (Murphy, Smith, Lindesay & Slattery, 1988) where there was a significantly higher four-year mortality for those who were depressed even when physical illness was controlled for. The same finding emerged in a study where elderly medical inpatients with depression were compared with nondepressed controls from the same population matched on age, functional status, type and severity of illness, and extent of disease (Koenig et al. 1989). In a fraction of these cases, the mortality may be due to suicide (Dorpat, Anderson & Ripley, 1968).

Interactions

Much of previous research on pain and depression has focused on two interactions between pain and depression: pain leading to depression, and depression secondary to pain (e.g., Gamsa, 1990; Banks & Kerns, 1996; Meana, 1998). As illustrated in preceding chapters, these may be incorporated within a larger framework of hypotheses about the possible relationships between pain and depression. Firstly, depression may be a correlate of pain. There are also dynamic interactions, as when depressive traits predispose an individual to pain, or when a depressive episode precipitates pain over the short run. Even when it has no causal role in pain, depression may aggravate or modulate pain intensity. Along similar lines, depression may perpetuate the duration or course of pain. Finally, depression may be a consequence of pain. The evidence for each of these six possible interactions is reviewed in the following sections. In addition, a special section is devoted to the notion of "pain as masked depression". Each of these interactions has unique and important implications for the treatment of depression (Joukamaa, 1994).

Depression as Correlate of Pain

Most investigations into the relationship between pain and depression report frequency data (as in epidemiological surveys) or else correlational data. Pain intensity is moderately correlated with depression (Tait, Chibnall & Margolis, 1990; Arnstein, Caudill, Mandle, Norris & Beasley, 1999) whereas pain duration is less so

(Kramlinger et al., 1983; Haley et al. 1985; Turner & Clancy, 1986). Philips and Jahanshahi (1985) found that neither duration nor chronicity of headaches varied significantly with depression, although people with more frequent headaches were more likely to be depressed. Even though Averill et al. (1996) recently reported that pain duration accounted for a significant portion of variance in depression scores, this amounted to less than 3% of the total variance.

Burns et al. (1999) studied a sample of 71 male recipients of workers compensation who had sustained musculoskeletal injuries. These patients had BDI scores that were moderately correlated with pain duration (r = .15) and significantly correlated with pain severity (r = .29). The correlation between pain and depression has been a subject of investigation in many types of pain, menstrual pain being of special concern. With menstruation occurs various hormonal and psychological changes including mood variability. This has sometimes been viewed as a reason for the higher rates of depression in women than men.

Bancroft, Williamson, Warner et al. (1993) found that in women with dysmenorrhea, menorrhagia or premenstrual syndrome, the severity of pain (particularly during the premenstrual phase) was related to the severity of depression. This was based on correlations between retrospective ratings of pain and depression. In a subsequent study (Bancroft, 1995), daily ratings of pain and depression were obtained for the duration of the premenstrual week and the days of menstrual bleeding in a sample of 201 women. Rank-order correlations revealed a significant association between pain and depression ratings premenstrually, r = .16, and during menstruation, r =. 37. This of course does not imply causation. In fact, the contribution of a third factor, menstrual bleeding, must be considered since it was correlated with depression in both these studies. Therefore, the depression associated with menstrual and premenstrual pain may be either moderated or enhanced by the contribution of concurrent physiological processes.

The association between depression and pain of abortion has also been studied (Belanger, Melzack & Lauzon, 1989). Subscale scores and total score on the McGill Pain Questionnairre (Melzack, 1975) correlated with depression at about r = .40 in this population.

One measure that has gained much credibility in pain measurement is observable pain behavior. With this as a predicted variable, the variance accounted for by depression often does not reach significance in those with rheumatoid arthritis (Anderson et al., 1988; Buescher et al., 1991; McDaniel et al., 1986) or in fibromyalgia (Baumstark et al., 1993; Buckelew et al., 1994). However, by semi-structured interviews and observations of patients in clinical settings, Turk and Okifuji (1997) obtained a correlation of .40 between depression and pain behavior in fibromyalgia. Depression as assessed by the CES-D added a significant 17% to the variance already accounted for by physical findings, physical capacity, and pain severity in this instance.

Using a prospective design, Kazis, Meenan and Anderson (1983) found no significant relationship between chronic pain of arthritis and depressive symptoms over a six-month period. However, Ferguson and Cotton (1996) reported a consistent linear relationship between pain and depression at five points in time over more than a year. Correlating these at one point in time, r = .54. This is similar to the correlation of .49 reported by Arnstein, Caudill, Mandle, Norris and Beasley (1999).

In the few between-groups designs, the relationship between pain and depression tends to be much weaker than in correlational studies. For example, Kerns and Haythornthwaite (1988) found no significant difference in pain severity among groups of nondepressed, mildly depressed, and depressed pain patients.

Depression Predisposing Pain

When depressive traits rather than depressive episodes are the cause of pain, then they are referred to as predisposing factors. Just as anxiety can be a state or trait, depression can be viewed as a trait -- as in the depressive personality disorder described in DSM-IV-TR (American Psychiatric Association, 2000) or in the work of Calfas, Ingram & Kaplan (1997). The notion of depressive personality traits culminating in pain has led some to adopt the term pain-prone personality. This invites debate about whether or not there is such an entity prone to pain by virtue of characterological features.

Among the traits clustered around depression is the tendency to devalue or blame oneself to the point of self-punishment. Blumer & Heilbronn (1984a) presented a psychodynamic view of the character of the pain-prone patient. As depicted in the following excerpt, this is a picture of a guilt-driven, self-sacrificing person who undergoes a transformation from "solid citizen" to chronic pain patient:

> Psychodynamically, the dramatic change from a prematurely responsible, independent, overly active and industrious individual to a passive-dependent suffering invalid, reflects the collapse of the "superhuman" counterdependent and counterpassive posture which had been adopted at an early stage. The patients often state they believed that they could do everything! Psychologic testing tells the inner story, of which the patients appear unaware.[6,12,13] Their basic attachment needs tend to be very marked, and needs to receive affection and to be cared for are often similarly enhanced. These basic "infantile" needs obviously have never been acknowledged by the patients, Their passive-submissive needs, to the extreme of masochism, are unique for this group,

and combined with their eagerness to please others in order to be accepted, results in relentless industriousness and self-sacrifice for the sake of the family. Anything socially unacceptable is guilt-provoking and is anxiously concealed and controlled. By increasing activity and work performance, their inner security and guilt had been soothed and a certain acceptance gained until the dilemma eventually became too painful. After a significant loss or disappointment, with or without the advent of a painful injury or ailment, a shift occurs which is drastic in its outward effect. It transforms the "solid citizen" into an invalid and heightens the same painful dilemma. The patient becomes passive, dependent and in need of care, but there is an enormous need to implicate a physical problem in order to maintain the ideal view of oneself (p. 797)

In a related formulation, Schafer (1994) borrowed the term "typus melancholicus" from Tellenbach's (1983) personality typology to explain a predisposition to migraine in some individuals. Also found in unipolar depressives, this personality type is characterized by oversensitive conscientiousness. According to psychodynamic principles, when the individual is unable or prevented from acting in this manner, s/he becomes overwhelmed by guilt, and this causes depression, which in turn leads to migraine in certain individuals. Personality tests of 127 migraine sufferers versus other groups confirmed the authors' hypothesis that migraineurs are similar to depressives, yet significantly different from healthy normals. Schafer is careful to point out that he is not suggesting a migraine personality, but that at least in some migraine sufferers, there are traits related to depression that increase the likelihood of a migraine attack.

One of the few studies to examine guilt and related features of depressed pain patients is that by von Knorring et al. (1983). They found that depressed patients who also had pain did not have greater guilt than their depressed pain-free counterparts.

Schmale (1972) contrasted depressive character styles with depressive affect and depression as a clinical syndrome. He stated that those who lack self-confidence and trust of others might develop a strong predisposition to experiencing helplessness and hopelessness. This in turn produces a somatic vulnerability which embodies symptoms such as pain.

One chronic pain syndrome that has often been attributed to psychological idiosyncrasies is phantom pain. It has been speculated that patients with this condition become vulnerable to pain especially if they have some premorbid personality features. Taking up this hypothesis, Sherman, Sherman and Bruno (1987) compared nearly 500 amputees with and without phantom pain on Rotter's (1966) locus of control scale. The locus of control scale measures the degree of one's perceived autonomy over life situations, and this has been commonly related to depression. Sherman et al. (1987) found that scores on this scale did not differentiate amputees with versus without pain nor did they relate to the intensity, frequency, or duration of pain. Two observations arise at this point. First, it is to be expected that loss of a body part will lead to grief, bereavement, loss of control and other feelings consistent with depression. It does not take premorbid personality traits to generate depression in such circumstances of disfigurement and dysfunction. Second, the depression in these cases is probably not responsible for pain. As much as a puzzle that phantom pain has remained, the weight of the evidence points to important neural substrates underlying this phenomenon.

A more modern investigation of the role of personality versus mood variables in pain has been made possible by the state-trait dichotomy in recent psychological instruments. Thus, Gaskin, Green, Robinson and Geisser (1992) utilized such instruments as the State-Trait Personality Inventory (Spielberger, Jacobs, Crane, Russell, Westberry, Barker & Johnson, Knight & Marks, 1979) and the Beck Depression Inventory to differentiate between affective states versus traits. A sample of individuals with chronic pain due to arthritis or fibromyalgia completed these questionnaires as well as the MPQ. Regression analyses of the data revealed that transient mood (e.g., depressive states) but *not* dispositional affect significantly predicted subjective pain report. This suggests that depressive traits are not significant predictors of pain.

Depression Precipitating Pain

Here, the issue is whether a depressive episode can trigger a separate and distinct episode of pain. For example, does depression pre-surgery increase the likelihood of pain post-surgery (as analogous to the anxiety literature where pre-surgical anxiety increases post-surgical pain)? This can best be ascertained by measures obtained repeatedly over a period of time.

In a short-span longitudinal study (Feldman, Downey & Schaffer-Neitz, 1999), 109 individuals with reflex sympathetic dystrophy completed daily diaries for pain and mood. Time-lagged within-subject analyses indicated that the previous day's depression did predict the current day's pain. However, the effect size was greater when the previous day's pain was used to predict the present day's depression. So, while there is a reciprocal effect of pain and depression, the contribution of depression to pain may be a secondary effect arising from helplessness and motivational deficits in dealing with the pain.

In another longitudinal study, herpes zoster patients were assessed for pain and psychosocial measures and then followed-up in interviews at three, five, eight, and twelve months later (Dworkin, Hartstein, Rosner, Walther, Sweeney & Brand, 1992). On questionnaire measures of depression, those who developed chronic pain scored higher than those who did not develop continuing pain at three months. However, nonparametric tests necessitated by the small sample sizes and heterogeneity of variance did not produce significant differences between these two groups of patients at initial assessment. This does not question the contribution of depression to post herpetic pain but it limits the extent of that contribution.

Perhaps, depression, by leading to inactivation and withdrawal, could result in physiological changes like deconditioning of the musculoskeletal system and that makes one more vulnerable to pain. Maybe certain behaviors too follow from depression, and these could increase the likelihood of pain, just as anger leads to certain consumptive behaviors. For example, the withdrawal that results from depression may be inconducive to getting appropriate social support or even medical and psychological care, and so pain is left untreated. The inertia of the chronic pain patient may make it difficult to seek out healthcare. But again, this does not mean that the withdrawal is a causative factor; it is more like an enabling factor.

Affleck, Tennen, Urrows and Higgins (1991) instructed rheumatoid arthritis patients to record their average daily pain intensity before retiring each night for a total of 75 days. After the first week, patients were administered a depression scale and a disability scale and every two weeks they were further examined for disease progression. It was found that 36% of the variance in pain intensity was explained by disease activity, disability and depression, the last two of these emerging as unique predictors of pain. The authors interpreted their results as meaning that depression at the start predicted pain in later days. However, this is no basis on which to infer causation or even temporal order. Depression measured during or at the end of the 75-day period of pain monitoring could have been correlated with pain in much the same way as depression in the first week predicted pain. In that case, all that could be suggested is a correlation between the two measures. Besides, the comparable contribution of disability scores to pain intensity suggests that a mediational model might be more accurate (as has been proposed in a few other studies).

Engel, Von Korff & Katon (1996) conducted a prospective study of 1059 enrolees in a health maintenance organization

(HMO) who consecutively presented at one of the participating clinics with back pain (including pain of thoracic and cervical spine). Three-to-six weeks after this visit, the patients were reached by telephone for a 30-minute baseline interview on various pain parameters, depression, disability, and sociodemographics. Depression was assessed by the Symptom Checklist-90, Revised (SCL-90; Derogatis, 1977), the 12 items on the depression subscale being rated on a 5-point Likert scale. For the next 11 months, computer-automated data from the HMO were used to determine the utilization and costs of health care services received in total or for back pain in particular. Multiple logistic regression analysis was performed to estimate odds ratios adjusted for age, gender, education, two-way interactions among these variables, and other predictor variables. This analysis showed that depression was only weakly predictive of back pain costs. If these costs are viewed as a proxy for pain and suffering, then depression can hardly be considered a strong precipitant of pain, at least in back and neck pain sufferers.

One study that utilizes a prospective design plus the statistical tool of covariance structural modeling to permit causal inferences about the interaction between pain and depression is that by Brown (1990). Because of its uniqueness and methodological innovativeness, this study merits extended coverage. Consent forms were mailed out to a pool of 744 adult patients diagnosed with rheumatoid arthritis for an average of about 3 years; of these, 387 (52%) agreed to participate. These participants were mailed a set of self-report measures every 6 months for 6 waves of data collection. Measures included the pain scale from the Arthritis Impact Measurement Scales (AIMS; Meenan, Gertman & Mason, 1980), a Visual Analogue Scale of pain intensity over the past 6 months, and the Center for Epidemiological Studies-Depression scale (CES-D; Radloff, 1977). The total number of participants completing the study was 243 (75% women and 25% men). Structural modeling was performed using LISREL-VII computer program (Joreskog &

Sorbom, 1985). Specifically, a series of three-wave, two latent-variable models were tested on the variance-covariance matrix with data from Waves 1,2, and 3, followed by a series of identical models tested using data from Waves 5,6, and 7 for the same panel of 243 subjects. Each model also possessed pairs of across-time correlated disturbances among repeatedly measured variables. Goodness of fit indices revealed that both the pain-to-depression model and depression-to-pain model fitted the observed data. However, to determine which model provided the best fit, each model was compared to the saturated and null models. For Waves 1, 2, and 3, both models were not significantly different from the saturated or null models. However, for Waves 5, 6, and 7, the pain-to-depression model did not fit significantly worse than the saturated model and fit significantly better than the null model, while the depression-to-pain model fit significantly worse than the saturated model and did not differ significantly from the null model. This led Brown to the conclusion that "only the pain-depression model both affords a more parsimonious representation of the data than the saturated model and maintains a comparable goodness-of-fit for Waves 5-6-7" (1990, p.132).

Depression Aggravating Pain

A number of early experiments have tested the responsivity of depressed individuals to noxious stimuli. In one of the earliest studies of this kind, Hall and Stride (1954) reported an increased threshold for heat pain administered to depressed patients, particularly those with endogenous depression. Merskey (1965) however found that compared to healthy normals, depressed patients had lower tolerance for pressure pain induced by an algometer. Overlooking the differences in modality of stimulation, this suggests that depression may reduce sensitivity to minimal levels of noxious stimulation but also reduce the maximum amount of pain an individual can endure.

In conceptualizing sensitivity, an important distinction must be made between sensory threshold and pain threshold. Von

Knorring and Espvall (1974) for instance found no significant difference between depressives and healthy controls in detection of electrical stimuli but significantly greater electrical pain threshold in the depressive group. More recently, Lautenbacher et al. (1994) carefully demonstrated that the increased pain threshold in depressives is not attributable to reaction time but to decreased pain sensitivity. Furthermore, they confirmed that this decreased sensitivity did not extend to non-noxious stimuli such as mere warmth, cold, and vibration.

The type of depression also seems to make a difference to pain sensitivity. Ben-Tovim and Schwartz (1981) found that electrical pain thresholds were higher in depressed patients with "emotional indifference" as compared to those without such a feature. Similarly, Bezzi, Pinelli and Tosca (1981) found that in a group of endogenous unipolar depressives, the "retarded depressives" had higher electrical pain thresholds than the "agitated depressives" or the healthy controls. This is also consistent with the observation by Von Knorring (1978) that depressed patients with psychotic symptoms had higher electrical pain threshold and tolerance (though not electrical detection threshold) than depressed patients without psychotic symptoms.

An important question that arises is whether the moderating effects of depression on pain represent an actual sensory-perceptual deficit or some kind of response bias. This takes the discussion into the domain of signal detection theory. One of the early investigations in this area was by Davis, Buchsbaum and Bunney (1979). Delivering random sequences of electrical stimuli to 66 patients with bipolar or unipolar depression, the authors saw evidence of a raised criterion for reporting pain as well as decreased sensitivity in a subgroup of depressed patients. Adopting a similar paradigm, Clark, Yang and Janal (1986) also found a stricter criterion for response to noxious heat in psychiatric patients (including depressives) but a decreased discrimination ability as well.

More recently Dworkin, Clark and Lipsitz (1995) used signal detection theory to examine responsivity to both painful and nonpainful heat stimuli. Twenty six patients with major depression and 15 with bipolar disorder (diagnosed according to DSM criteria) were compared to 32 normal controls. It was found that depressives had higher response criteria at all levels of stimulation, but discriminability was dependent on stimulus intensity: at higher intensities of noxious stimulation, depressives had poorer sensory discrimination than controls, this difference vanishing at lower levels of noxious stimuli. Bipolar subjects did not differ significantly from depressives but they did have more elevated response criteria than controls at lower levels of noxious stimulation. Based on these and earlier results, the authors concluded that depression attenuates responses to pain by lowering sensory discrimination as well as increasing the stoical bias against reporting pain.

In general, at least in the context of experimentally induced pain, depression attenuates rather than aggravates the pain. This attenuation is related to changes in the perception and labeling of pain unlike comparable investigations of schizophrenics where there appears to be an overall somatosensory deficit (Lautenbacher & Krieg, 1994). The perceptual change may be related to hormonal and other mechanical processes during depression; the labeling is likely due to motivational characteristics in decision-making. The very few studies not reporting attenuation of pain in depressives are limited by such problems as small sample sizes, the presence of only mild levels of depression, and a restricted range of noxious stimuli.

Further research is needed to extend the present findings to clinical pain. Unfortunately, clinical pain does not permit the degree of internal control required of signal detection theory experiments. In such clinical investigations, it will not be sufficient to show that depressed pain patients have more pain than nondepressed pain counterparts since the directionality of influence remains unknown. More convincing evidence might emerge if it were shown that pain patients who become depressed for reasons other than the pain end up with more pain than they began with.   This temporal sequence of events coupled with changes in select variables would allow a stronger test of the hypothesis that depression attenuates pain.

Depression Perpetuating Pain

Depression has also been considered a possible reason for the perpetuation of pain.   Unlike the aggravation of pain which refers to an escalation in intensity, the perpetuation of pain pertains to its extension over time.

The psychoanalytic tradition has several references to pain perpetuated by depression and the defensive need for self-punishment.   Freud had recognized some individuals' apparent need to be ill as a possible result of guilt and feelings of worthlessness (Freud, 1937, 1940).   Luborsky and Auerbach (1969) observed that episodic stomach pains and migraine headaches were among the somatic symptoms sustained by feelings of helplessness.   The dominant theme here is a compensatory process in which pain makes up for depression.

An interesting case study has been provided of a 26-year old woman with a history of miscarriages, and other physical symptoms like headaches, pain, and general malaise that served as self-expiation for feelings of worthlessness associated with depression (Schmale, 1972).   In the course of psychoanalytic therapy, the patient spent much time ruminating about her unworthiness as a daughter, wife, parent, and nurse. She revealed a long-standing pattern of trying to please others while denying her own needs. The pain and discomfort she experienced during her pregnancies became a way of making up for feelings of inadequacy and depression. When she finally managed to have her first child, she developed new confidence and joy, but this was soon undermined by the baby's crying which left her with a sense of feeling underappreciated. Months later, she had to have a painful cyst removed from her mouth, and the familiar theme of self-punishment reappeared when she viewed the pain as the price for her recently increased self-esteem on having her first child. Even if one does not subscribe to the pscyhodynamic interpretation of this pain as rooted in an unresolved oedipal conflict, it is easy to see how the pain makes up for feelings of unworthiness, and is thereby perpetuated by the depressive cognitions of the patient.

In contrast to the compensatory principle promulgated by psychoanalysts, learning theory suggests that reinforcement plays a pivotal role in the maintenance of pain by depression. (Banks & Kerns, 1996; Romano & Turner, 1985). In the present context, one possibility is that depressive behaviors of helplessness elicit help which in turn promotes pain behavior.

Pain Causing Depression

Like the depressive antecedents of pain, the depressive consequents of pain deserve discussion. It is hardly surprising that prolonged pain or physical stress of any kind would result in depression; this fits with the theory of learned helplessness. Yet, psychiatric views of the nature and etiology of depression have often ignored this possibility even in chronic pain patients. This may be due to the psychodynamic tradition in psychiatry that has been inclined to locate the cause of affective disturbance in childhood conflicts. As portrayed by von Brauchitsch (1975):

> Yet, the fact that physical illness produces depression - does not fit into our psychiatric concept of the nature and etiology of depression. Physical illness should produce anxiety because of the potential threat to survival. The central feature of melancholia, however, is diminished self-esteem traceable to disturbances of early psychosexual development, or more specifically an introverted rage reaction caused by the narcissistic loss of an highly ambivalently cathected superego introject. It is impossible to explain how such a reaction can be

triggered off by physical illness. The conventional dynamic model of melancholia is therefore not applicable (p. 73)

In reviewing the family practice records of patients undergoing treatment for depression, Widmer and Cadoret (1978) found a rise in pain complaints during a seven-month period prior to the diagnosis of depression. This increase was absent during a seven-month period three years before the diagnosis of depression. Therefore, the more likely scenario was that pain led to depression rather than vice versa.

As mentioned earlier, daily diaries for pain and mood in reflex sympathetic dystrophy showed that the previous day's pain significantly predicted the present day's depression (Feldman, Downey & Schaffer-Neitz, 1999). Previous day's depression also did predict the current day's pain, but the effect size was smaller. The Brown (1990) study detailed earlier used a prospective design coupled with structural equation modeling to show that there is more support for depression as a consequence of pain than the reverse.

Pain as a Symptom of Depression (Masked Depression)

The concept of pain as a depressive symptom is really a variation of the idea of pain secondary to depression. Epidemiological research cited earlier has indicated that in about a third to two-thirds of depressives, pain is a symptom (Lindsay & Wyckoff, 1981; Magni, Schifano & Deleo, 1985; Singh, 1968; Spear, 1967; Von Knorring et al. 1983; Wells et al. 1989). The pain in these cases tends to be mild-to-moderate in magnitude and may not be chronic but it seems to be a *part of* the depressive presentation.

Some scholars have extended this to a view of "pain as masked depression" or pain as a depressive analogue, a way of legitimizing the depression. Blumer and Heilbronn (1984b) argue this point as follows: "If depressive symptoms were merely secondary to the pain, as the critics state, by what miracles can antidepressant drugs abolish the chronic pain in many of our patients, when used as for major depressive disorders?" (p.406). The mechanism by which antidepressants drugs work is still a matter of some debate as will be discussed later but there is no reason to dismiss the possibility that pain can be a symptom of depression.   Most psychometric tests of depression have not incorporated pain as an item but at least for a subset of patients, this might be worth considering.

A related idea is that pain is a cover up for depression.   The depression may be buried deep or close to the surface.   In the former, there may be complex psychological conflict or severe trauma that may withhold the depression from being expressed except as conversion disorder.   In the latter, social desirability factors may dissuade the individual from communicating depression.   For example, Rosenbaum (1982) has argued that pain patients may be reluctant to show affective disturbance out of conformity to the role of the medical patient and out of fear of being labeled as a psychiatric or psychological case.   Others (e.g., Joukamaa, 1994) have related masked depression to alexithymia. Coined by Sifneos (1973) alexithymics are limited in their ability to verbalize feelings, have an impoverished fantasy life, use actions to avoid conflict, and rarely dream or cry.   Consequently, their affect is expressed in the form of physical symptoms or trivial environmental details.

In a treatise on masked depression, Lesse (1974) has identified a myriad of "masks" for depression -- from pain and a variety of psychosomatic symptoms to substance abuse, impulsive sexual responding, antisocial behavior, sadism and masochism, compulsive work, and even accident proneness.   These behaviors and illnesses are regarded as alternate pathways for the resolution of depression or some psychological conflict.   This is supported by clinical observations over a 17-year period (Lesse, 1983).

The related idea of pain as a mere symptom of depression has been articulated by von Brauchitsch (1975).   He speaks of phantom limb patients "who in practically every respect qualified as agitated depressions. I would like to stress that observation because it implies that, at least in these cases, pain is not a depressive 'equivalent' but merely one of the symptoms of depression" (p.76).

Blumer & Heilbronn (1984b) remark "We have offered the parsimonious view that pain without peripheral cause stems from a muted mental agony ... akin to depression" (p.406). They add: "We have evaluated over the past 20 years, some 2000 chronic pain patients. Clinical evaluation of the patients and their families, assessment of their life histories, utilization of psychologic tests, and the study of biologic markers increasingly provided the empirical facts contributing to our formulation of the pain-prone disorder...It was only over the past 6 years that we recognized the pain-prone disorder as a variant of depressive disease" (p. 405). Others have also gone along with the idea that only a mask separates depression from chronic pain. However, as discussed in the section on mechanisms, there are alternate explanations for symptom overlap and there is declining evidence of common biological markers for these two conditions. Besides, the physiological basis of pain is an arousal mechanism, whereas that for depression is usually the opposite: a deactivation and slowing down of functions. This questions the idea of a common origin for depression and pain.

In a study designed to test the masked depression hypothesis, Van Houdenhove, Verstraden, Onghena and De Cuyper (1992) compared four groups of patients receiving mianserin in a double-blind placebo-controlled trial: group A (nonorganic chronic pain plus depression), Group B (organic pain plus depression), Group C (organic pain without depression) or Group D (depression alone). As expected, an antidepressive effect emerged for all except group C, but the effect was most pronounced in group D. However, there was no change in pain scores, not even in Group A which was regarded as a "masked depression" group. Had the pain in this group of patients been the byproduct of depression, an antidepressant effect should have been accompanied by an analgesic effect. The absence of such a finding led the authors to reject the hypothesis of masked depression in patients suffering from chronic idiopathic pain.

That chronic pain is masked depression or a variant of depressive disease has come to be widely regarded as a mistaken view. The mistake seems to have arisen primarily out of nosological confusion and crude measurement techniques. More discussion of this point can be found in the works of Gupta (1986), Pincus and Williams (1999), and Roy, Thomas & Matas (1984).

Miscellaneous Interactions

Mention should also be made of a few related formulations or variants of the above interactions. One is the "scarr hypothesis" (Fishbain, Cutler, Rosomoff & Rosomoff, 1997). This is the postulation that depressive episodes increase the probability of depression after the onset of pain. This is akin to the idea of pain as "masked depression". It also echoes diathesis-stress theory which will be evaluated in the next section.

Also, it is likely that more than one of the above interactions may operate in any single patient. For example, depression might aggravate or perpetuate pain and that in turn might intensify or perpetuate depression. This particular form of reciprocal interaction is recognized in many other areas of psychosomatic medicine, and it warrants consideration in the context of pain too.

Most studies cited earlier have tested single or unidirectional hypotheses of the link between depression and pain. One of the few tests of multiple hypotheses about pain-depression interactions was carried out by Lindsay and Wyckoff (1981). They asked 226 patients about the order of onset of pain and depression. It was ascertained that far more patients (38%) reported that depression came after pain than those who said the depression preceded the pain (12%), but the majority (50%) claimed a simultaneous onset of the two. These findings are generally in the same direction as back pain patients' recollections of the age of onset of their pain and depression (Atkinson, Slater, Patterson, Grant & Garfin, 1991). There were more instances in which the first depressive episode came after the chronic pain (58%) than instances in which the first depressive episode came before the chronic pain (42%). In only 15% of the latter group was the recalled onset of depression no more than two years before the recalled onset of pain. The authors interpreted this to mean that primary depression was rarely a cause of the pain. However, one should be mindful that this study utilized retrospective reports, and it is best to guard against attaching too much weight to them. In conjunction with the other studies discussed earlier, they do, however, help shed light on the old issue of how pain and depression are linked.

As can be seen, the question should no longer be whether depression causes pain or pain causes depression. For one thing, this is an oversimplification of the multiple ways in which pain and depression can interact. Patients differ in the interactions that apply to their condition, so research must turn to the question of which patient is characterized by what type of interaction between pain and depression. In his survey of this research domain, Lipowski (1990a) estimates that in about 50% of comorbid pain and depression, the two states develop concurrently; in 40% of the cases, depression follows pain, leaving the remaining 10% in which depression precedes pain. This seems to be consistent with most other empirical investigations into this topic. Fernandez, Clark and Rudick-Davis (1999) emphasized new methods for further distinguishing patients according to the particular type of interaction between pain and depression. Borrowing from other areas of psychology, this entails concurrent self-monitoring of both pain and depression over a period of time. Alternatively, longitudinal studies extending over years can provide an even wider window into the onset of episodes or diagnoses of depression in relation to pain.

Mechanisms

Some scholars have proposed a common etiology for chronic pain and depression. This may have origins in ancient medicine where the same treatments for physical pain were often prescribed for mental anguish. Opium once used by the Egyptians for pain relief was later put to use by the Greeks in treating melancholia. In fact, until the late 18th century, the terms melancholia and hypochondria were used in reference to the same phenomena (Lund, 1994). The nosological confusion seems to have persisted to the present day as pointed out by Roy et al. (1984) who lists several terms (e.g., "unique depressive disorder", "atypical depression", "mixed depression" and "depression without depression") that have been used to justify the presence of depression in pain patients.

Genetic Family Studies

The idea of a shared mechanism for depression and chronic pain received an impetus from research on first degree relatives of pain patients. For example, Katon, Egan and Miller (1985) reported that 30% of a sample of chronic pain patients had first degree relatives with an affective disorder. Specifically, depressive disorders have been reported in 65% of the first degree relatives of patients with chronic pain (Schaffer, Donlon & Bittle, 1980). However, there is also evidence to the contrary. Recent research that carefully combined interviews, medical records, and the administration of the SCID (Spitzer, Williams, Gibbon & First, 1992) in a sample of women with chronic pain revealed no differences in family histories between those with and without depression (Dowhrenwend, Marbach, Raphael & Gallagher, 1999).

It is insufficient to rely on family history alone. Studies of identical versus fraternal twins and adoptees are needed before confidence can be expressed in the notion that the depression of pain patients runs in families. Rarely are the concordance rates for identical twins much more than 50%. Even then, it is hard to exclude the possibility that social and environmental factors might explain the concordance of depression between the proband and other family members (Andreasen, 1987).

The position that chronic pain and depression share a common etiology or that one is a variant of the other weakens when one considers the quite different courses taken by these two conditions.   Whereas chronic pain usually persists for several years, major depression is typically episodic. Perhaps dysthymia rather than major depression would be a closer parallel to chronic pain.   Is dysthymia a more common form of depression in pain patients than is major depression?   Data from Large (1986) suggests that this is indeed the case, dysthymia being diagnosed in 28% of pain patients referred for psychiatric evaluation, as opposed to only 8% of the same sample receiving a diagnosis of major depression.   Data from more than 3000 inpatients in consultation-liaison psychiatry services at two metropolitan general teaching hospitals in Australia revealed more comorbidity of somatoform disorder and dysthymia than any of the other depressive disorders (Smith, Clarke, Handrinos & Dunsis, 1998). The earlier cited data of Fishbain et al. (1986) also confirmed this disparity, with 23% of pain patients having dysthymia compared to 6% with major depression.

Symptom Overlap

Assertions about shared etiology may also be rooted in a misattribution of sleeping difficulties, psychomotor retardation and other vegetative symptoms to depression. These same symptoms are equally likely to arise from prolonged pain (Sherman, Sherman & Bruno, 1987). Quality of sleep at night has been shown to be related to amount of pain in the preceding day while also influencing pain the next day (Affleck, Urrows, Tennen & Higgins, 1996). Pain patients classified as good versus poor sleepers differed in pain intensity as well as depression (Pilowsky, Crettenden & Townley, 1985) and the relationship between sleep and depression appears to be over and above that of pain and depression (Nicassio & Wallston, 1992). Similarly, there is ample evidence that chronic pain produces limitations in ambulation, body care, and home management (e.g., Dionne & Turcotte, 1992). As emphasized by Fifield, Reisine and Grady (1991), these structural barriers have an independent effect on depression in pain patients.

Common Biological Markers

Apart from the similar clinical presentation, there are other points of convergence between depressives and chronic pain sufferers. At least in idiopathic pain patients (where there is no organic basis for the pain), certain biological markers of depression have been claimed. These include shortened latency of rapid eye movement in sleep EEG (Blumer et al. 1982), hypercortisolemia (Ward et al. 1992), and low concentrations of melatonin in serum and urine Beck-Friis, 1983).   Such observations have led von Knorring (1989) and von Knorring and Ekselius (1994) to assert a common pathogenetic mechanism for chronic pain and depression. However, it must be noted that these so-called biological markers of depression are far from definitive. They do not necessarily characterize all or even most depressives, and the replicability of these findings is unstable.   The presence of such correlates in chronic pain patients is even less, often confined to patients with so-called idiopathic pain syndrome.

In an elaborate investigation of the hypothesis of common biological markers, Van Kempen, Zitman, Linssen and Edelbroek (1992) selected several biochemical parameters supposedly involved in depression and explored their presence in chronic pain patients *without* depression.   The reasoning is as follows: if depression and chronic pain involve the same biological mechanisms, then patients with chronic pain should share these same biological markers of depression. These markers included serotonergic activity (the enzyme monoamine oxidase-B in thrombocytes, platelet serotonin and thrombocyte phenosulfotransferases), markers of central noradrenergic activity (plasma levels of 3-methoxy-4hydroxy-phenylethylene glycol and its sulfate conjugate) markers of cholinesterase activity (plasma cholinesterase, and urinary phenylacetic acid) and plasma cortisol. Participants were carefully screened to form a group of 34 patients with chronic pain aged 30-60 years, without substance abuse, psychiatric disorders needing intervention, or other medical problems such as renal, hepatic or cardiac disorders. With the exception of a positive correlation between pain and monoamine oxidase-B, *no other correlation turned out significant.* This challenges the notion of shared etiology for chronic pain and depression. Furthermore, this same study found that in a 16-week trial of amitryptiline, about a third of the patients received at least 50% relief from pain. However, there was no relation between treatment outcome and any of the biochemical parameters described earlier.

A review of the literature by Lund (1994) supports the suggestion by Van Kempen et al. (1992) that chronic pain and depression are neurochemically more different than alike. The classical monoaminergic neurotransmitters (serotonin, dopamine and noradrenaline) were compared between chronic pain and depression, as were cortisol, substance P, Beta-Endorphin and Somatostatin. The research was found to be *inconclusive if not contradictory* on the issue of neurochemical similarity between chronic pain and depressed patients. With the exception of serotonin reductions, the only chemical that seemed to hold some interest as a common marker was somatostatin. Somatostatin-like immunoreactivity was reportedly reduced in the CSF of patients with major depression (Molchan, Lawlor, Hill, Martinez, Davis, Mellow et al. 1991; Traskman-Bendz, Ekman, Regnell & Ohman, 1992) as well as in chronic pain patients (Urban, France, Bissette, Spielman & Nemeroff, 1988). In any case, these studies are too few in number and too preliminary to justify any reliable inferences.

Beutler, Daldrup, Engle, Oro'-Beutler, Meredith and Boyer (1987) investigated the possible role of β-endorphin in reductions of pain and depression during Gestalt psychotherapy. This kind of therapy was successful in producing a decline in depression and (to a lesser extent) pain in women with rheumatoid arthritis, but the correlation between pain and β-endorphin levels was modest at best and that between depression and β-endorphin levels was in the range of −0.33 to +0.39. It was concluded that pain and depression are relatively independent phenomena and that the reduction in the latter is not mediated by changes in β-endorphin levels.

Common Personality Traits

It is no less plausible to consider psychological markers of depression in chronic pain as it is to speak of shared biological markers. Several personality traits found in major depressives have also been reported in patients with idiopathic pain, 50% of the latter showing the same discriminant function as the former (von Knorring, Almay & Johansson, 1987). Conversely, there is another 50% who do not share the same personality traits as depressives. Idiopathic pain patients reportedly have raised scores for muscular tension, social desirability, psychasthenia, socialization, and inhibited aggression but low scores for impulsiveness, monotony avoidance, indirect aggression, and suspicion. On the bases of this characterization, von Knorring (1989) has argued "Thus, it seems reasonable to assume that chronic pain syndromes and depressive disorders may occur with an increased frequency in subjects with roughly the same personality traits, probably leading to an increased vulnerability towards the two syndromes" (pp. 36-37). However, such an inference is rushed and tenuous in view of the possibility of other medical conditions characterized by such traits. In other words, this subset of traits may not be uniquely shared by chronic pain and depression. High muscle tension, social desirability bias, nervousness, suspiciousness, and inhibited aggression are also descriptive of various anxiety disorders and some personality disorders. Moreover, it is quite plausible that the above features such as muscular tension, inhibited aggression, and monotony are a direct offshoot of the persistent pain itself rather than the result of a depressive personality. It is debatable if these features constitute personality traits, but even if they did, it should be pointed out that chronic pain can change people's personalities (Garrin & Leavitt, 1983; Sherman, Sherman & Bruno, 1987; Sternbach, 1968; Weisenberg, 1975; Vittengl, Clark, Owen-Salters & Gatchel, 1999).

Cognitive Styles

Related to the concept of personality are cognitive styles. These may also be viewed as schemas -- cognitive structures that govern the screening, coding, assimilating, and interpretation of information. Deficits in one or more of these stages of information processing have been identified in depressives but how this relates to the chronic pain population is only just beginning to be systematically studied.

Pincus, Pearce and McClelland (1995) have examined the information processing biases in depressed pain patients as compared to individuals with clinical depression alone. The pain patients were presented with words such as "guilty" and "shameful" that were consistent with a depressive schema, and words such as "suffering" and "disabled" that were associated with an illness schema. Results showed that pain patients had a negative recall bias to the latter but not the former schema. It was concluded that depressed pain patients differ from clinically depressed individuals in their concept of depression. Similarly, selective memory tasks suggest a qualitative difference in schemata between those with chronic pain and those with depression (Edwards, Pearce, Collett and Pugh, 1992).

Cognitive Distortions

Related to the above information processing deficits is Beck's (1967, 1976) cognitive model of depression in which distorted thinking is responsible for depression. Thus, chronic pain patients may evaluate themselves as worthless, their pain as devastating, and their functional ability as severely compromised. Research does suggest a role of such cognitive distortions in the depression associated with chronic pain (Ingram, Atkinson, Slater, Saccuzzo & Garfin, 1990; Ingram, Slater, Atkinson & Scott, 1990; Philips, 1989; Smith, Peck, Milano & Ward, 1988). These studies show that in depressives, negative thoughts predominate over positive thoughts, they occur in automatic fashion, and they are organized into self-schemas. These distortions are far more apparent in depressed pain patients than in pain patients without depression (Lefebvre, 1981).

Diathesis-Stress Theory

An important hallmark of psychopathology and psychosomatic medicine that may have explanatory value for pain-depression research is diathesis-stress theory. Long used to explain schizophrenia and mental illness, diathesis is any personal characteristic (biological or psychological) that increases the likelihood of developing a disorder. The stress or stressor is an environmental stimulus or life event that compromises the individual's coping resources. The combination of a specific vulnerability to a disorder plus any kind of unpropitious event is what culminates in the particular disorder. Applying this to chronic pain, Banks and Kerns (1996) suggest that an inherent vulnerability to depression (as manifested in negative schemas) when activated by the stress of chronic pain, leads to depression. Primacy is given to the organismic variable instead of the situational trigger. This notion has been criticized by Williams (1998) on the grounds that the focus is on a flaw within the patient. It is certainly conceivable that some patients carry a proneness to depression that governs their response to chronic pain or other forms of stress, but can most depression in chronic pain patients be attributed to such a diathesis? No gene has been discovered for depression, and there is a lack of á priori prediction about how early development determines later depression. Given the high comorbidity between chronic pain and depression, the pain itself could make a unique contribution to depression. Banks and Kerns (1996) acknowledge such a possibility but only in the context of a reciprocal model in which pain escalates depression without being responsible for it.

It is difficult to test diatheses-stress theory because of its teleological quality: we can infer depressive vulnerability once depression occurs, but not prior to it. We know what percentage of the population has depression but we do not know what percentage of the population is vulnerable to depression; no doubt, the latter exceeds the former. Many people may not yet have developed depression, but (according to diathesis-stress theory) they may fall prey to it when struck by calamitous life circumstances. This resembles the AA view of alcoholism in which a sort of latent alcoholism supposedly resides in some people waiting to be "released" by the particular situation in which they would resort to uncontrollable drinking.

If we turn to point prevalence data, DSM-IV-TR estimates about 5% of the general population as having major depression. This is nowhere near the rates of major depression in the chronic pain population, which, by conservative estimates, average about 40% (Davidson et al., 1985; Haley et al., 1985; Shafer, 1980). Even if the 3% dysthymics in the general population are added, the disparity between community and chronic pain samples remains very wide. Perhaps, a better estimate of the percentage vulnerable to depression is the lifetime prevalence rate. In the general population, this is 13% for major depression and 6% for dysthymia (according to DSM-IV) as compared to more than 50% in the chronic pain population (Katon, Egan & Miller, 1985). This means that the risk of depression in chronic pain sufferers is nearly three times that in the general population. At best, diathesis-stress theory can barely explain half the cases of depression in the chronic pain population. On the other hand, there is a strong possibility that nearly two-thirds of the cases of depression in chronic pain are the result of something other than an inherent vulnerability to depression, probably something peculiar to the pain and its psychosocial impact on the individual.

Perhaps, stress may outweigh diathesis in the development of chronic pain. After all, when pain becomes chronic, the patient may have to adjust to the need for frequent medical consultation, changes in physical activity, occupational retraining, and interpersonal support. In the terminology of Holmes and Rahe (1967), the life change units become a measure of the stress level. There is a particular quality of "loss" in the chronic pain experience much like the sense of loss that characterizes depression. This loss is not confined to such tangibles as income and physical function but extends to a loss of self-esteem, loss of social life, and loss of interest. Collectively, the losses and life changes must be an important force in the culmination of depression.

Life Interference

In keeping with the view that stress and change are important proximal determinants of depression in pain patients, a wave of research has addressed the problem of life interference from pain and injury. Mohamed, Weisz & Waring (1978) found that when compared to patients with depression, patients with both pain and depression had significantly more interpersonal problems, especially with their spouses, their families, and spouse's family. The authors viewed these marital and familial problems as mediators between pain and the somatic presentations in depression. Comparing various sociodemographic and pain-related variables of interest, Averill et al. (1996) found that work status accounted for most of the variance in depression among multidisciplinary pain clinic referrals. Although this amount was just under 5%, it does suggest that disruption in employment does play a role in the depression experienced by chronic pain patients.

In a longitudinal study, Ferguson and Cotton (1996) assessed pain, sleep patterns, social activity, and overall disability as possible predictors of depression in 81 Australian women with rheumatoid arthritis. These measures were obtained every 3-4 months at five successive points in time. Data were analyzed by hierarchical regression. Apart from the strong association between pain and depression, it was found that higher levels of overall disability were associated with higher levels of depression six months later. The Time 1 measures of depression, social activity, and an interaction between social activity and sleep accounted for significant increases in the variance of depression at Time 5. This is partially consistent with longitudinal data from Nicassio and Wallston (1992) that led to the conclusion that "although sleep disturbance appears to be aggravated by prior pain, its existence may contribute to subsequent mood disturbance" (p.519). When aggregated, these findings point to life interference as an important mediator in the link between pain and depression.

Older people provide another case in point. Their increased susceptibility to depression is not simply a function of the years that have passed. Instead, depression in the elderly has been shown to be largely due to the life-interfering effects of pain and illness. These include restricted mobility, erosion of self-image, and dependency on others (Aneshensel et al. 1984; Fenton, Cole, Engelsmann & Mansouri, 1994; Turner & Noh, 1988). In their interviews of survivors of 200 deceased community residents (all over age 65) Moss, Lawton & Glicksman, (1991) found an increase in pain from 37% at one year before death to 66% at one month before death. Lower levels of pain were associated with less depression, but what is more striking is that the increase in pain was related to a decline in quality of life over the last year. By implication, any increased depression in aging pain patients is probably attributable to declining vitality, deterioration in vocational, social and familial relations, and overall difficulties with daily living.

A compelling test of whether life interference is indeed a mediator between pain and depression is possible using structural modeling. As conceived by Joreskog (1978), this approach embeds factor analysis within the path analytic tradition to come up with an idea of the relative strength and directionality of relationships among variables.   The first study to employ such methodology in testing the role of life interference between pain and depression was by Rudy et al. (1988).   The authors proposed a mediational model with four factors or latent variables: pain severity, life interference, self-control, and depression.   Pain severity was operationalized with scores from the MPQ, the MPI, and two weeks of hourly self-monitoring.   Life interference was operationalized with scores from the social, work, and family interference scales of the WHYMPI (Kerns, Turk & Rudy, 1985); self-control was operationalized with scores from the life control and problem-solving scales of the WHYMPI and the Internal subscale from the Multidimensional Health Locus of Control (Wallston, Wallston & DeVille, 1978).   Depression was measured by the Beck Depression Inventory (Beck, et al. 1961) and the Depression Adjective Checklist (Lubin, 1965).   Against a null model of no covariation among these variables, a mediational model was tested in which pain severity was hypothesized to increase life interference and decrease self-control both of which would culminate in increased depression.   Results revealed that the mediational model fitted the data well while the null model did not.   All hypothesized coefficients among the latent variables were statistically significant except for the direct path between pain and depression.   Moreover, 68% of the variance in depression was explained by the three predictors.   However, the partial correlation between pain and depression was near zero when either life interference or self-control was controlled for.   This suggests that there is hardly a direct link between pain and depression and that life interference and loss of self-control are indeed the mediators between pain and depression.

If disability and interference in day-to-day life is pivotal in depressive reactions to pain, then it follows that functional restoration should decrease depression in pain patients.   This has been demonstrated in patients with low back pain (Owen-Salters, Gatchel, Polatin & Mayer, 1996) and in a sample of patients with spinal injuries (Mayer, Gatchel, Kishino, Keeley, Capra, Mayer, Barnett & Mooney, 1985). These authors' findings that improved physical capacity and functional restoration led to improved mood in pain sufferers do indicate that physical disability and impairment are part of the life interference that is responsible for depression in pain sufferers.

Helplessness

An important ingredient in the depressive process is the individual's perception of help. Circumstances perceived to be beyond control lead to cognitive, motivational, and behavioral deficits that portray an individual who has given up. This has been termed learned helplessness (Seligman, 1975) and it has significant affective consequences. Particularly when the individual develops stable, global, and internal attributions about lack of control, depression is the likely outcome (Abramson, Seligman & Teasdale, 1978).

It is not surprising that chronic pain refractory to treatment and persisting for months and years brings about learned helplessness. This would be characterized by beliefs that the pain is beyond control, an erosion in efforts to deal with it, an apparent inertia, and a high probability of depression. Using regression analyses, it has been shown that chronic pain is related to helplessness (Engle, Callahan, Pincus & Hochberg, 1990) and that pain and helplessness predict depression (Tayer, Nicassio, Radojevic, & Krall, 1996). When residualized change scores between pretreatment and posttreatment were the outcome measure, hierarchical regression confirmed that changes in helplessness accounted for a significant increase in variance in pain even after depression scores were controlled for (Burns, Johnson, Mahoney, Devine & Pawl, 1998).

More recently, path analysis has been used to test this mediational model of pain, helplessness, and depression (Nicassio, Schuman, Radojevic & Weisman, 1999). Participants were 122 individuals with fibromyalgia lasting an average of 12 years. They were assessed on Helplessness and Internality subscales of the Rheumatology Attitudes Index (Callahan, Brooks & Pincus, 1988), the latter tapping into beliefs of personal controllability over the illness.   Additionally, depression, pain and disability were assessed.   As predicted, the greater the pain, the greater the depression, r = .55.   After removing the effects of age, pain and disability jointly explained 34.5% of the variance in depression. Pain and disability were positively related to helplessness and negatively related to internality but while helplessness significantly predicted depression, internality had no independent relationship to depression.   The mediational model as a whole explained 47% of the variance in depression.

Another path analytic study of 126 outpatients at pain clinics (Arnstein, Caudill, Mandle, Norris & Beasley, 1999) examined self-efficacy (the converse of helplessness) as a mediator in the pain-depression relationship.   Results confirmed that in addition to a significant relationship between pain intensity and depression, disability was a mediator between the two, accounting for 32% of the explained variance in depression.   However, when self-efficacy was added to the model, it attained a significant path coefficient with depression (β = -.31), while the path between disability and depression lost significance.   In addition, self-efficacy also predicted disability.   This led the authors to come up with a new model in which both pain intensity and self-efficacy contribute to disability and depression in chronic pain patients.

The earlier-cited study by Rudy et al. (1988) used structural modeling to demonstrate that self-control (together with life interference) mediates the link between pain severity and depressive symptoms.   Self-control was operationalized in terms of how much control patients had over their lives, how much they felt able to solve problems in the preceding week, and their internal locus of control over health.   These are positively related to feelings of self-efficacy and inversely related to feelings of helplessness.

Reinforcement Contingencies

Learning theorists have explained that the mechanism of depression may involve loss of positive reinforcers in their environment (e.g., Bloschl, 1975; Buchwald, 1977) or else the loss of effectiveness of these reinforcers (Costello & Lazarus, 1972). In the context of chronic pain too, there has been recognition of the reinforcing effects of certain life events on depression (Romano & Turner, 1985; Banks and Kerns, 1996).

Kerns and Haythornthwaite (1988) found that groups of depressed, mildly depressed, and nondepressed chronic pain patients tended to differ more on instrumental activities, coping skills, and support from significant others than they did on pain severity. Moreover, their reduction in depression with treatment paralleled improvements in daily activities and support from others. As the authors conclude, pain is not a sufficient condition for depression. Rather, like many depressed people, depressed pain sufferers have diminished social rewards and face increased interference with the performance of pleasurable activities. This lends support to a cognitive-behavioral mediational model of pain and depression.

Assessment of Depression in Pain Sufferers

The psychological assessment of depression has relied greatly on self-report depression inventories and structured interviews. This section will provide a glancing review of such questionnaires and interviews that have been applied to the pain population. As many of these methods have been extensively reviewed within the depression literature, what is offered here are some guideposts for selecting appropriate methods for the pain population.

Depression Scales

The Hamilton Rating Scale for Depression (Hamilton, 1960, 1967) was the first well-known psychological instrument for assessing depression, other scales often using it as a validating standard. Different versions of this semi-structured interview have appeared, of which the 21-item version has been the most popular. More recently, a paper-and-pencil forced choice format has been adopted, giving rise to the Hamilton Depression Inventory (HDI; Reynolds & Kobak, 1995). In general, the Hamilton scales are designed to quantify severity of depression. Compared to other depression inventories, the HDI uses multiple probes for each symptom, thus assuring greater confidence in the measurement of depression (Fernandez, 1998a). After considering issues of clinical utility, Rabkin and Klein (1987) concluded: "In summary, the HSRD remains the preferred measure of the two for assessing depressive severity, if the means are available to use either. In the absence of sufficient clinical resources, or for some specific practical or research question, the BDI may serve as an acceptable approximation of the HSRD" (p. 65). In the context of chronic pain, the Hamilton scales have successfully discriminated between low back pain patients and depressed patients without pain (Davidson et al. 1985).

The Beck Depression Inventory (BDI; Beck, Ward, Mendelson, Mock, & Erbaugh, 1961) has surpassed the HDI, with reportedly more than 2000 empirical studies using or evaluating it (Richter, Werner, Heerlin, Kraus, & Sauer, 1998). The BDI is a 21-item self-report scale. Each item consists of four graded statements which are ordered according to increasing depressive symptomatology. The range of scores is from 0 - 63. The recommended cutoff scores are < 10 for absence of depression, 10-18 for mild to moderate depression, 19-29 for moderate to severe depression, and >29 for severe depression (Beck, Steer & Garbin, 1988). For patients referred to a multidisciplinary pain clinic, mean total score on the BDI = 15.82, S.D. = 9.93, range = 1 to 50 (Averill et al. 1996). The BDI has been found to be reliable and valid not only in the general population of depressives (Beck et al., 1988) but also in the chronic pain population. Novy, Nelson, Berry and Averill (1995) have demonstrated its factorial validity, in particular, evidence for a single higher-order depression construct that makes it meaningful to use the total depression score in this instrument. Due to the problem of overlapping symptomatology between chronic pain and depression, Peck, Smith, Ward and Milano (1989) proposed the omission of eight somatic-related items from the BDI. Others have computed separate mean scores for a subgroup of items (14-21) measuring primarily somatic symptoms versus those (items 1-13) that pertain to cognitive symptoms (e.g., Crisson, Keefe, Wilkins, Cook, & Muhlbaier, 1986).

The Center for Epidemiological Study – Depression Scale (CES-D; Radloff, 1977) is a 20-item self-report scale originally meant to assess depression in the general population. Each item is a question about the frequency with which a particular symptom was experienced in the past week, ranging from 0 (not even once a day) to 3 (daily). Four items are reverse-scored. The total score, ranging from 0 to 60, indicates the frequency of depressive symptoms currently experienced. Internal consistency has been in the high range ($\alpha = 0.85 - 0.92$) in the general population and patient samples -- irrespective of age, gender, race, and geographic location (Radloff & Teri, 1986). In a sample of 126 chronic pain patients administered the CES-D, the α coefficient was equally high at 0.90 (Arnstein, Caudill, Mandle, Norris & Beasley, 1999). Validity has also been established in chronic pain patients but as mentioned earlier, some correction is needed for overlapping symptoms between chronic pain and depression. Some scholars (e.g., Blalock, DeVellis, Brown & Wallston, 1989; Brown, 1990) exclude four items pertaining to disease pathology irrespective of depression. These are "I felt that everything I did was an effort", "My sleep was restless", "I felt hopeful about the future", and "I could not get going". Others (e.g., Magni et al., 1990; Turk & Okifuji, 1994) raise the minimum cutoff for depression from 16 to

19 when using the CES-D to assess depression in chronic pain sufferers.

The Zung Depression Scale (Zung, 1965) is a self-report questionnaire with 20 items to be rated on a 4-point Likert-like scale. It was used in some early studies of pain and depression (e.g., Ward et al. 1982). When administered to a group of patients with chronic pelvic pain, none turned out clinically depressed (Ehlert, Heim & Hellhammer, 1999). It does not seem to discriminate well between depression and anxiety (Mendels & Weinstein, 1972) and is less reliable than the HSRD (Hedlund & Vieweg, 1981). Because of its emphasis on somatic-vegetative signs, it tends to overestimate depression in patients with severe chronic pain (Estlander, Takala & Verkasalo, 1995).

The Depressive Adjective Check List (DACL; Lubin, 1965) is a list of 32 adjectives to be self-rated as applicable or not applicable to oneself. Tasto (1977) has reported that the DACL is reliable but not sensitive when differentiating moderate from severe levels of depression.   Rudy et al. (1988) reported a correlation of 0.42 between this measure of depression and scores from the BDI.

The Montgomery-Asberg Depression Rating Scale (Montgomery & Asberg, 1979) has 10 items, each scored on a 7-point scale. A clinician is supposed to complete the scale on behalf of the patient. The scale's greatest promise is as a measure of clinical change in drug trials. Krishnan et al. (1985) found that the Hamilton Depression Scale and Montgomery-Asberg scale discriminate between patients with various types of depression and chronic pain.

In the interest of brevity and simplicity, Snaith et al. (1971) picked 10 of the most frequently endorsed items from the Zung and added two more to create the Wakefield Depression Inventory (WDI). In one of its few instances of use in the pain population, the WDI appeared to lack discriminability between depressed versus nondepressed headache sufferers (Philips & Jahanshahi, 1985).

Depression Subscales

The Symptom Checklist 90 (SCL-90; Derogatis, 1977) and SCL-90-R (Derogatis, 1983) are 90-item checklists of symptoms to be rated on a 5-point Likert-like scale. Thirteen of the items belong to the depression factor. These pertain to mood and loss of interest, self-blame, hopelessness, worthlessness, suicidality, and a couple of somatic symptoms. This scale has been used in the chronic pain population (e.g., Engel, Von Korff & Katon, 1996) and seems to be sensitive to treatment-induced changes. However, Rabkin and Klein (1987) view this as part of a general halo effect on all subscales of the instrument.

The Profile of Mood States (POMS; McNair, Lorr & Droppleman, 1981) is a list of 65 mood-related adjectives rated on a 4-point scale in terms of amount/frequency. One of the six subscales is called depression-dejection. Reliability and validity coefficients are high. One observation, however, is that the scores over time are not always in agreement with scores averaged over multiple points in time (Rasmussen & Jeffrey, 1995).

The Institute of Personality and Ability Testing Depression Scale (Krug & Laughlin, 1976) is a global measure of depression comprising 40 items related to low energy, guilt, resentment, suicidal ideation, boredom, and hypochondriasis. Marbach and Lund (1981) have administered it to facial pain patients but found no difference in their depression scores as compared to normals.

The Hospital Anxiety and Depression Scale (HADS; Zigmond & Snaith, 1983) is worthy of mention even though it has not been widely applied to pain patients. Unlike most of the other depression inventories, the HADS was developed in a population of physically ill patients. It is therefore particularly suited to the chronic pain population.

Structured Interviews and Miscellaneous Depression Instruments

There are two interview-based methods that are particularly useful in the differential diagnosis of depression. One is the Schedule for Affective Disorders and Schizophrenia (SADS; Endicott & Spitzer, 1978) and the other is the Structured Clinical Interview (SCID; Spitzer, Williams, Gibbon & First, 1992). They require considerable time to complete, but are likely to be more diagnostically accurate than self-administered tests. Both have been used occasionally on pain patients (e.g., Dworkin, Clark & Lipsitz, 1995).

Several other depression instruments do make occasional appearances in the pain literature. As listed by Roy, Thomas and Matas (1984), these include the Checklist of symptoms, Cronholm-Ottoson depression scale, Levine-Pilowsky depression scale, Middlesex questionnaire, Depression scale of the Institute of Personality and Ability Testing, and the Hoffer-Osmond Diagnostic Test. Readers interested in those and related instruments are referred to other existing reviews of depression assessment, in particular the books by Marsella, Hirschfeld and Katz (1987) and Nezu, McClure, Ronan, and Meadows (2000) respectively.

Measurement Issues

Diagnosis

Studies have revealed that depression is often undiagnosed or misdiagnosed by physicians. In medical outpatients, the error rates are about 50% (Moffic & Paykel, 1975; Knights & Folstein, 1977), while for medical inpatients, they are even higher (e.g., Schwab, Bialow, Clemmons & Holzer, 1967). This may be related to somatization and the comorbidity of depression with other disorders. More than half of primary care patients with depression or some psychiatric disturbance also present with somatic complaints (Bridges and Goldberg, 1985). These authors demonstrated that in 48% of such cases, physicians misdiagnosed the problem (usually as a physical ailment), though when the symptoms were purely affective, the correct diagnosis was reached in 98% of the cases.

Errors of omission and commission in the diagnosis of depression may also depend on who the diagnostician is. The pain patient who gets to see a psychologist, psychiatrist or mental health professional is more likely to have depression diagnosed accurately than when seen by a physician in general practice.

There are also differences of opinion about nosological systems and diagnostic criteria to use. Blumer and Heilbronn contend: "There are obvious reasons why no psychiatric disorder has ever been discovered through statistical methods. What we recognize as a disorder distinct from all others is invariably a complex entity, presenting in many variations and degrees of severity, defying mathematical formulations" (1984b, p.405). The many different labels and differential weighting of criteria for depression have already been discussed in the introduction to this chapter.

DSM and the Problem of Overlapping Symptoms

Many of the DSM-listed symptoms of depression are also independently indicative of chronic pain. For example, sleep disturbance, motor slowing, anergia or loss of energy, appetite and weight change, are to be expected in patients suffering from chronic pain *even if they are not depressed.* For example, low back pain patients awaiting neurological evaluation had physical complaints that are also characterstic of depression (Crisson et al. 1986); this has been observed in many other medical conditions too. Without the requisite cognitions and subjective affect, it would be precarious to attribute such complaints to depression. It should be noted that DSM-IV criteria require that diagnoses of major depression not be made in instances when these symptoms are due to a general medical condition.   Therefore, strictly speaking, chronic pain patients should never be diagnosed with major depression if the depression is in any way related to the pain.

BDI, CES-D

Many psychometric tests of depression are also not equipped to differentiate between primary depression and depression secondary to chronic pain or medical illness.   The Hospital Anxiety and Depression Scale (Zigmond & Snaith, 1983) is one of the few tests of depression normed in a medical population.   On the other hand, the Beck Depression Inventory, the Hamilton Rating Scale for Depression, and the Zung Self-Rating Depression Scale generate a unidimensional score based on somatic, cognitive, and affective features of depression.   In the case of chronic pain patients, this total score tends to be elevated above that for depressives because of the many somatic symptoms arising directly out of pain and illness (De Vellis, 1993; Williams & Richardson, 1993). Numerous studies of medical populations consistently show high endorsement of somatic items on depression scales and an overdiagnosis of depression.   But because the depression scales were rarely normed on medical populations, it can be difficult to interpret the total scores in terms of how much reflects depression and how much reflects symptoms of medical illness (Mayou & Hawton, 1986).

To correct for the endorsement of somatic items by nondepressed patients, higher cutoff scores have been recommended when using depression scales in medical populations (Cavanagh, 1983; Bridges & Goldberg, 1984).   The cutoff scores for major depression can be raised in the case of chronic pain too.   Turk and Okifuji (1994) recommend a minimum score of 19 instead of the usual 16 when using the CES-D for assessing depression in chronic pain sufferers.   Other researchers (e.g., Blalock, DeVellis, Brown & Wallston, 1989; Brown, 1990) have chosen to drop four items from the CES-D because of their connection to disease pathology irrespective of depression. These include the items "I felt that everything I did was an effort", "My sleep was restless", "I felt hopeful about the future", and "I could not get going". Similarly, in the case of the BDI, Calfas, Ingram and Kaplan (1997) have suggested omitting eight somatic-related items when assessing depression in similar populations. These items pertain to sleeping difficulties, fatigue, reduced appetite, weight loss, concerns/worries about health, reduced interest in sex, enjoyment doing things, and effort required to do things. The resulting shorter version of the BDI enhances discriminability of state-depressed, trait-depressed and nondepressed individuals.

The confounding of somatic-behavioral and cognitive-affective symptoms of depression may be responsible for the greater prevalence rates of depression in chronic pain populations as compared to depressed populations. Most studies of the chronic pain group have not adopted higher cutoff scores for depression and therefore are more likely to label these patients as depressed. Most studies also appear to have ignored DSM stipulations that major depression is not the proper diagnosis if it is secondary to a medical condition.

Another source of false positives in depression inventories is that the cognitive items may not be specific to depression (Boyle, 1985). Instead, these items may be associated with other psychiatric conditions such as the anxiety disorders which overlap with depression in symptomatology. They may even occur as part of the normal adjustment process (Gottlib, 1984). One promising solution for the specific problem of confounding between anxiety and depression seems to be available in a new instrument called the Depression Anxiety Stress Scales (Lovibond & Lovibond, 1995).

MMPI

Measures of depression in pain patients have often been derived from the MMPI which has found widespread application not only in psychiatric populations but also in the pain population (Keller & Butcher, 1991).   However, the MMPI was never intended to differentiate normal chronic pain patients from those with psychological complications like depression (Sherman, Sherman & Bruno, 1987). This leads to the increased probability of inferring depression in pain patients when it may simply be a normal part of the adjustment process to chronic pain (Pincus, Callahan, Bradley, Vaughan & Wolfe, 1986). Additional caveats have been pointed out in a critical review of the MMPI (Helmes & Reddon, 1993) and in reviews of the MMPI as used in pain patients (Deardorff, 2001; Turk & Fernandez, 1995).

Cultural Appropriateness

Assessing depression is an enterprise where culturally appropriate methods have often been overlooked. The ensuing errors are even more pronounced when the test-takers are pain patients who are themselves subject to a myriad of cultural influences (Rollman, 1998). Thus, handing a questionnaire to a pain patient is hardly the ideal approach to assessment, least of all when the patient is culturally unaccustomed to that format of disclosure. Two case studies illustrate this point.

A single case study of a Turkish immigrant to Switzerland, illustrates the culturally appropriate tools needed to probe and understand depression associated with pain in this patient (Yilmaz & Weiss, 2000). This includes overcoming linguistic barriers as well as seeking information from family members. Another case study (Frances & Kroll, 1989) reports on a Hmong woman who had pain in the muscles and joints plus depression possibly complicated by her refugee status in the U.S., the death of her husband and concerns about her 17-year old daughter. The case illustrates the multiplicity of issues that can contribute to depression and the cultural shaping of depressive symptomatology. This requires interviewing not just the patient but family members, and enlisting the support of other people from the community whom the patient identifies with. Even an appropriately translated psychological test may miss the intricacies and nuances of depression in these scenarios.

Diagnostic Documentation

The timing of the pain and depression needs to be carefully ascertained before inferences can be made about causality. As pointed out by Banks and Kerns (1996) point out, the search for depression in chronic pain patients usually begins well after the pain has begun, because the pain must persist for six months before it is deemed chronic. Similarly, for depression, there is a minimum of two weeks before it is diagnosed as "major". This means that when a diagnosis of major depression is made just after an injury or painful episode, the depression actually began at least two weeks prior thus making it an antecedent instead of a consequent of the injury or pain. Similarly, if a diagnosis of major depression precedes a diagnosis of chronic pain by two weeks or even two months, that does not mean that the former is an antecedent of the latter because at least six months would have transpired since the pain began.   This issue can be further dissected to make a distinction between *point of diagnosis versus point of onset*. There is nothing magical or momentous that happens after two weeks' depression that transforms it into something "major", nor is there an upheaval after six months of pain that makes it qualitatively different from pain with a shorter history.   These are merely arbitrary cut-offs and the point of diagnosis is not the point of onset for either major depression or for chronic pain. The upshot of all this is that it becomes even more difficult than previously assumed to make inferences about the temporal (let alone, causal) relationships between depression and pain based on diagnostic documentation alone.

Retrospective Data

Proper identification of the type of interaction between pain and depression is imperative if these problems are to be effectively treated.   The few studies exploring temporal order and other dynamic interactions between pain and depression have relied primarily on patients' recall of events or else on diagnostic history as recorded in medical charts.   Patient recall is affected by the obvious limits of human memory and by patients' limited understanding of constructs like depression. Chart records obviate the need for long-term recall and the diagnoses contained therein are less open to dispute since they were made by clinicians. However, as mentioned earlier, chart entries tend to record the onset of diagnosis but not necessarily the onset of the problem. If pre-diagnostic information is recorded, it is usually based on patients' recall.

A more definitive approach to tracking the onset of depression in relation to pain is by daily monitoring over an extended period of time.   Such an approach also corrects for the temporal instability in mood disturbances such as depression. For example, prevalence rates for depression in a sample changed from 44% to 72% over a 12-week period (Gallagher, Moore & Chernoff, 1995). This suggests that point-in-time measures are likely to be less reliable than repeated measures over time.

Affleck, Tennen, Urrows and Higgins (1991) illustrate how daily self-monitoring can be used in combination with other periodic assessments to obtain pain, depression, disability, and disease progression scores in rheumatoid arthritis patients. For 75 days, these patients recorded their average daily pain intensity before retiring each night. A week into the monitoring, patients were administered a depression scale and an arthritis impact scale. Every 2 weeks, patients were examined by a rheumatology nurse for joint swelling and other disease activity.   The concurrent measures allowed bivariate analyses of the data over time. Had depression been monitored in the same time series as pain, it would have been possible to discern the temporal relationship between the two. Similar approaches have been used to study the relationship between stress and headache (Kohler & Haimerl, 1990; Levor, Cohen, Naliboff, McArthur & Heuser, 1986).

The concurrent monitoring of depression and pain over an extended period of time can greatly illuminate the interplay between depression and pain. By training the patient to record events as they happen and wherever they happen, data collection becomes convenient as well as ecologically valid (Fernandez & Beck, 2000). Hence, this procedure has recently come to be known as Ecological Momentary Assessment (Stone & Shiffman, 1994). It now incorporates the use of technology ranging from wristwatches (Litt, Cooney, & Morse, 1998) to palm-top computers (Stone, Schwartz, Neale, Shiffman, Marco, Hickcox, Paty, Porter, & Cruise, 1998). Such devices can also be used to promote instantaneous and naturalistic data collection on depression and pain.

Pain Measurement

Much has been faulted in the way depression is measured, but criticisms are also in order for pain measurement. In most pain-depression studies, the adequacy of pain measures has been taken for granted. One self-report measure of pain that has been frequently used in this area is the McGill Pain Questionnaire or MPQ. Despite its long history in pain assessment (having also been translated into several languages), the MPQ is in need of refinement. Recently uncovered problems of factor instability and classification ambiguity now raise doubts about the validity of scores on the sensory, affective and evaluative scales of this instrument (Fernandez & Towery, 1996; Towery & Fernandez, 1996; Fernandez & Boyle, 2002; Holroyd et al. 1996; Torgerson & BenDebba, 1983).

Another concern is about how a diagnosis of chronic pain is reached. Ordinarily, this is based on a temporal yardstick of six months. Many studies lump together patients diagnosed with chronic pain irrespective of the *chronicity* of their pain. A patient with a history of six years' pain is quantitatively and qualitatively different from one with six months of pain, and this difference can greatly influence the measures of depression in these patients. Some studies merely report the average chronicity of pain as part of a table of demographic and descriptive features of the sample. This is better than leaving it unknown, but it still leaves the problem of considerable error variance due to such heterogeneity. As aptly stated by Roy (1986), a diagnosis of chronic pain is an inadequate indicator of the severity of pain.

The diagnosis of pain is also affected by changing nosology. There has been a transition from the DSM-II diagnosis of pain as a psychophysiological disorder, to the DSM-III concept of psychogenic pain disorder, to the DSM-III-R category of "somatoform pain disorder" to the DSM-IV diagnosis of "pain disorder" further subclassified as "psychological", "secondary to medical condition", "combined" or "unspecified". As pointed out by Verma and Gallagher (2000), quite different inferences are reached about the relationship between chronic pain and depression, depending on which of these definitions is adopted.

In his review of five years' literature on pain and depression, Roy (1986) found that most studies used single measures of pain, such as number of hours of pain over a day, or percent of time that the pain was felt. Such durational and frequency measures were common. However, this ignores the intensity of pain, let alone measures of disability and function. The lack of commonality in measures has also hindered reviewers' ability to compare and integrate findings across the literature (Roy, 1986). More comprehensive measures of pain can enhance comparability of results across studies as well as increase the likelihood of finding select relationships between pain and depression.

One classification system that stands out in its comprehensiveness is the IASP taxonomy (Merskey, 1986). It allows a diagnosis of pain with reference to five axes: anatomical site, physiological system, etiology, temporal pattern, and intensity.

Other Diagnoses

The linking of depressive events to pain must also be placed in the perspective of many other developments in the patient's life. For example, Atkinson, Slater, Patterson, Grant & Garfin (1991) found that the onset of substance abuse preceded pain in 81% of back pain patients. Together with the 58% of cases in which they found that the first episode of major depression occurred after the onset of pain, the authors concluded that substance abuse is far more likely than depression as a precursor of chronic back pain.

Other Conditions, Other Symptoms, Overall Morbidity

Finally, it is also important to keep in perspective that pain may be only one of multiple symptoms in a disease where depression occurs. The depression may be related to the overall morbidity of the disease. For example, Hawley and Wolfe (1988) found a close relationship between depression and progression of rheumatic disease over a three-year period. Likewise, in a condition like diabetes, neuropathic pain may be responsible for only part of the depression since patients also face dehydration, hunger, breathing difficulties, visual deterioration, nephropathy, and even gangrene. Research so far has not separated the contributions of pain from the other sources of morbidity in an illness. In their review of depression in the medically ill, Rodin, Craven and Littlefield (1991) reported consistent evidence of a relationship between "illness severity" and depression in the medically ill, particularly when subclinical levels of depression were measured. No doubt, pain is one of the most common presenting symptoms in patients and possibly the most aversive one too, but its contribution to depression must be assessed in relation to other symptoms responsible for the overall morbidity of an illness.

Treatment of Depression in Pain Sufferers

Psychological Treatment

Despite the prevalence and prognostic implications of depression in chronic pain, it has been pointed out that most depressed chronic pain patients do not receive treatment for depression, those who do receive treatment are most likely to receive medication instead of psychological intervention, and those medicated are more likely to be prescribed narcotics than antidepressants (Sullivan, Reesor, Mikail & Fisher, 1992).   Yet, psychological options for the treatment of depression have been extensively researched and applied in non-pain patients.   In a couple of Australian university hospitals, psychological management has been shown to be the mainstay of treatment for depressives, though not without the addition of antidepressants   (Smith, Clarke, Handrinos & Dunsis, 1998).   These scholars found that comparable percentages of major depressives were referred for psychological intervention as were recommended   antidepressant   medication   (about   75%),   but psychological intervention was recommended twice as often as medication in the case of dysthymia, and four times as often in the case of adjustment disorder with depressed mood.

Psychodynamic therapy. One of the earliest schools of psychotherapy is founded on Freudian psychoanalysis and psychodynamic therapy. As described earlier in this chapter, psychoanalysts regard depression as a reaction to loss that is real, imagined, or symbolic.   As in cognitive therapy, appraisals are given considerable importance in the etiology of depression. Arieti (1962), for example, distinguishes between "self-blaming versus a demanding form of depression called "claiming" depression. Each originates from a different genre of appraisals. The former results from attributions of sin or misdeed to the self, followed by self-blame and punishment. The latter results from high expectations of others which when not met lead to pleas for help and messages of dependency.

The point of departure between psychodynamic therapy and modern cognitive therapy is with regard to how these appraisals operate and how they ought to be corrected. Psychoanalysts (e.g., Arieti, 1962; Lesse, 1962; Spiegel, 1960) suggest that the abovementioned cognitions are relatively unconscious and symbolic of deeper ideation. For instance, a suicidal attempt might be a message: "I should do to myself what you should do to me, but you are too good to do it" (Arieti, 1962, p. 404). The psychoanalytic approach is not to openly contest these deep-seated appraisals. Instead, the therapist who invariably becomes a "dominant other" to the patient initially goes along with the patient's thinking in the service of rapport and transference. As Lesse puts it, this is ego-supportive therapy in which the therapist takes on the role of the "strong, all wise, all giving, all forgiving, protective paternal substitute" (1962, p.413).

Only after positive transference has been achieved can the therapist begin the task of correcting faulty appraisals. This change is achieved by bringing the unconscious appraisals to awareness by insight rather than instruction. Thus, free association and dream analysis are interspersed within a relatively unstructured therapeutic exchange. Once a measure of insight has been achieved, the therapist gradually encourages alternate forms of thinking and behavior, while slowly withdrawing from his/her role as paternal substitute or dominant other.

Despite the differences noted, it should be underscored that the psychodynamic approach is fundamentally cognitive in its focus, in that self-statements are subjected to interpretation. How they are interpreted of course is a matter of debate, the psychoanalysts often emphasizing the symbolic. The reliance on insight, however, is an approach that is shared by some current-day cognitive therapists who refer to their work as "guided discovery" or "collaborative discovery". Furthermore, psychoanalysts do engage in the gradual shaping of attributions and statements much as in cognitive therapy.

There are hardly any data on the efficacy of psychoanalytic therapy for depressed pain patients. This is partly because this school of therapy was at its heyday prior to the advent of behavior therapy in the 1960's. The concept of depression as a comorbid problem with pain did not come till much later, and the recognition of chronic pain as a problem itself did not reach the fore of the health professional community till the 1970's. The few studies of psychoanalytic treatment of depression may not stand up to the methodological standards of the present but they do suggest a positive outcome. For example, Lesse (1962) reported that 82% of 180 severely depressed patients showed remission of depressive symptoms and resumption of vocational and social responsibilities following a combination of antidepressant medication and psychoanalytic therapy. The former lasted a minimum of 3 weeks primarily to stabilize patients, while the latter lasted anywhere from two months to a year.

Cognitive reappraisal and restructuring. The primacy of cognitions in emotion (as explained in Chapter 1) has led to the idea that emotions and affective disturbance can be treated by changing cognitions (Beck, 1976; Ellis, 1962). Also known as cognitive reappraisal, this approach has gained much currency in the treatment of depression by psychologists as well as psychiatrists.

Contrasting this approach with psychodynamic therapy, Beck (1991) explains that the idiosyncratic meanings people attach to events do not revolve around esoteric themes of sexuality but around vital social issues such as success or failure, acceptance or rejection etc. Furthermore, these cognitions are highly accessible to consciousness.

Depressives are inclined to make several classes of cognitive errors or distortions, e.g., overgeneralization, dichotomous thinking, selective abstraction, and arbitrary inference. These may have originated as controlled thoughts, then turned into automatic thoughts, and finally organized into broad networks of knowledge called schemata. The task in cognitive therapy is to straighten out this kind of thinking through rational disputation or the search for counterevidence. For example, an individual might interpret chronic pain as a sign that s/he is doomed to a life of invalidism and abandonment. This might be challenged by (i) pointing out that the individual is catastrophizing or exaggerating and lacks logical bases to make such a prediction (ii) marshalling counterevidence from other patients who have remained functional despite chronic pain (iii) turning to authoritative sources such as medical opinion. If, however, the client's ideation turns out to be supported, coping self-statements may be employed to assist him/her to adapt as much as possible to an unpleasant reality. Reappraisal and coping statements work best under collaboration instead of didactic methods. This may be time-consuming because it requires discovery and debate of various propositional statements if not the reconstruction of underlying schemas that drive these statements in an automatic fashion.

Research on chronic pain patients shows that they do tend to have cognitive distortions of the kind mentioned above and that these distortions are related to depressiveness in those with low back pain (Lefebvre, 1981) rheumatoid arthritis (Smith, Christensen, Peck & Ward, 1994) and other pain syndromes. Moreover, it has been demonstrated that pure cognitive interventions do have an ameliorative effect on this depression (Turner & Jensen, 1993). This positive outcome can extend to the restructuring of core beliefs or underlying schemas as found in pain patients with personality disorders (Young, 1999).

Behavior modification. As already explained, the behavioral model of depression asserts that depression is largely a function of consequences. These consequences include loss, absence, or reduction in rewarding events and/or an increase in unpleasant events. Such events may be brought on by the environment or by the individual. Behavior modification of depression, therefore, relies on changing individual behavior in conjunction with restructuring the environmental stimuli.   One picture of an unrewarding lifestyle might be that of an individual who has acquired a pattern of social withdrawal, physical inactivity, and overwork.   This individual's routine may be altered through the use of activity schedules that incorporate social engagements, exercise, and weekends out of town.   Because the desired behaviors are intrinsically pleasant, they can be shaped to increase in inverse relation to the unrewarding behaviors.   This basic principle has been successfully applied in pain patients to increase uptime and healthy behaviors at the expense of downtime and illness behaviors (e.g., Fernandez & McDowell, 1995).

However, a reservoir of other behavioral techniques awaits transfer from the literature on depression treatment. For example, Azrin and Besalel (1981) have summarized successfully implemented operant conditioning techniques such as behavioral contrast, overcorrection, and stimulus control for the control of depression.   Lewinsohn, Sullivan and Grosscup (1980) have drawn upon assertion training and time management.   Others (e.g., Gotlib, 1984) have emphasized the value of self-reinforcement in addition to sampling of external sources of reward.   This derives from Bandura's (1977) idea that an individual is always able to reward himself/herself even if not rewarded by others; therefore, this resource should be tapped into when the environment itself may be lean on rewards.

Experiential and emotive therapy.   Mayer (1975) emphasized the importance of allowing if not encouraging feelings in the psychotherapeutic treatment of depression.   She especially warned of those who inhibit feeling by medication or by psychological defense mechanisms.   "Such patients cannot be helped by psychotherapy unless and until the emotional barrier can be broken down" (p. 354). Through the safe and controlled release of pent-up affect such as depression, patients can find relief from distress and then achieve cognitive reorganization.

Beutler et al. (1987) engaged chronic pain patients in a highly focused abreactive form of psychotherapy based on Gestalt principles. This form of therapy was presented within an ABA design where the first A was a baseline of 4 weeks, B comprised early, middle and late treatments each lasting 3 weeks, and the return to A was at follow-up 4 weeks later. The patients were six women with pain and other symptoms associated with rheumatoid arthritis; they were not on any psychoactive medication, steroids or narcotics. The patients participated in such Gestalt techniques as the "two chair" dialogue through which they verbally and physically expressed their anger toward an imagined significant other in an attempt to achieve some resolution of relevant conflicts. The authors were operating on the assumption that unresolved anger lay at the bottom of depression and chronic pain. The outcome of this intervention was an improvement in both depression and pain. The former underwent a progressive decline from baseline to follow-up. The latter did not show a consistent linear decline from session to session but mean postsession pain levels were uniformly lower than those at presession.

It should be acknowledged that of late there has been some wariness about catharsis as a method of dealing with emotional disturbance such as depression. This stems from the fear that such an approach might lead to reinforcement of emotional expression without an appropriate cognitive shift or a shift to more adaptive behaviors.   Such a risk exists primarily when abreaction is attempted in an uncontrolled setting without the proper supervision of a highly trained therapist. As von Btauchitsch (1975) has pointed out, ventilation or abreaction is also contraindicated when the patient has secondary gain for depressive complaints and related symptoms.

Exercise.   The beneficial effects of exercise on psychological functioning have been investigated in more than a thousand studies many of which were reviewed by Folkins and Sime (1981) and Taylor, Sallis and Needle (1985). A recent review by Tkachuk and Martin (1999) found evidence for the benefits of exercise in specific conditions such as depression.

Basically, this review of 14 experimental or quasi-experimental studies of clinically depressed individuals revealed no report that exercise was ineffective, a consensus that aerobic exercise was superior to placebo, and a consensus that exercise compared favorably to individual psychotherapy for depression. The benefits typically emerged within five weeks of thrice weekly supervised sessions of aerobic activity or nonaerobic exercise of low to moderate intensity 20-60 minutes in duration. Furthermore, these benefits are maintained for up to a year, especially if regular exercise is continued. Such exercise is also more cost-effective than conventional treatments for depression (Freemont & Craighead, 1987).

It should be added that human movement may not only combat the psychomotor retardation of depression but may also serve a cathartic function when used as a medium for expressing emotion. Such movement-oriented techniques have been developed under the general rubric of expressive therapies. A recent volume by Weiner (1999) reflects the resurgence of interest in this approach as a complement to the talk therapies, and offers ideas for adaptation to the affective needs of pain sufferers.

Pharmacological Treatment

Considerable research has been invested in the development of drugs for combating depression. Such medications have become highly favored treatments for the depressed with or without pain. Known as antidepressants, these medications supposedly achieve their effects by altering neurotransmitter activity.

Depression is related to serotonin levels, and CNS serotonergic neurons are intimately involved in nociception. Some depressed individuals may also have abnormal levels of other biogenic amines e.g., norepinephrine. The ratio of serotonin to norepinephrine may predict depression and furthermore, pain. While serotonin potentiates the analgesic action of endorphins, raising the threshold of pain, norepinephrine inhibits endorphin action, lowering the threshold of pain. Antidepressants regulate the balance between serotonin and norepinephrine to varying degrees. For example, doxepin exerts most of its effect on norepinephrine whereas fluoxetine selectively acts on serotonin. In any case, the altered balance between these two neurotransmitters seems to alleviate depression and to some extent pain. The antidepressants most investigated in research on pain and depression are the tricylics. This class includes doxepin, amitryptiline, clomipramine, and imipramine.

There are four major classes of antidepressant medication. The first consists of Monoamine Oxidase Inhibitors (MAOIs). These are reversible or irreversible inhibitors of norepinephrine and serotonin catabolizing enzyme monoamine oxidase. They hinder the circulation of harmful pressor amines and reduce the nonspecific action of biogenic amines released from the nervous system and adrenal glands.

Tricyclic antidepressant agents (TCA's), so-named because of their three-ring structure, are competitive or reversible reuptake inhibitors of noepinephrine and serotonin. Inhibition of reuptake increases the concentration of the neurotransmitter in the synapse and extends the available time for the neurotransmitter to bind with receptors. The ratio of the reuptake of norepinephrine to serotonin depends on the particular TCA. Desipramine, for example, blocks reuptake of norepinephrine more so than serotonin, whereas clomipramine blocks reuptake of serotonin more so than norepinephrine.

Heterocyclic antidepressant agents (HCAs) do not have a three-ring structure but they are also competitive reuptake inhibitors of norepinephrine and serotonin. They are sometimes referred to as second-generation agents. Finally, selective Serotonin Reuptake Inhibitors (SSRIs) inhibit the reuptake of serotonin only. In doing so, they increase the availability of serotonin.

These antidepressant medications have been primarily used to treat depression, and bipolar disorder, and most controlled trials of these medications have been performed on depressed patients with no physical comorbidity (Kathol, Katon, Smith et al. 1994). A large database from two major psychiatry services revealed that antidepressants were prescribed to 75% of patients with major depression, 46% of dysthymics, 21% of those having adjustment disorder with depressed mood, and 47% with depressive disorder not otherwise specified. Yet, of those with both pain and major depression, only 14.5% received antidepressants (Smith, Clarke, Handrinos & Dunsis, 1998). An examination of the charts of 1145 patients seen at Beth Israel Hospital Pain Management Center in Boston Massachusetts between January 1993 and June 1994 revealed that only about 25% received antidepressant medications (Richeimer, Bajwa, Kahraman, Ransil & Warfield, 1997). However, the efficacy of these medications is not clear because of the lack of a separation of depressed from nondepressed pain patients in relation to separate effects on pain and mood.

In order to picture the main ways in which antidepressant medications are hypothesized to benefit pain sufferers, a 2x2 matrix can be constructed (as shown in Table 3). Along this matrix, there are two groups of pain patients (depressed vs. nondepressed) and two possible actions of antidepressant medication (analgesic vs. mood-elevating). The four cells thus formed cover the four possible outcomes of mood change and pain relief.

Table 3
*Predicted Effects of Antidepressants on Depressed vs.
Nondepressed Pain Patients*

		PAIN PATIENTS	
		Depressed	Not Depressed
ANTIDEPRESSANT MEDICATION	Analgesic Effect	Little	None
	Mood-altering Effect	Much	None

Given the premise that antidepressants are designed to alter mood rather than abolish pain, it would appear that:

1. Pain patients who are depressed derive little analgesic effect from antidepressants.
2. Pain patients who are depressed derive much mood-elevating effect from antidepressants.
3. Pain patients who are not depressed derive no analgesic effect from antidepressants.
4. Pain patients who are not depressed derive no mood-elevating effect from antidepressants.

These four hypotheses can be evaluated on the basis of research on antidepressants in the pain population. The inferences that emerge can collectively shed light on the mechanism of action of antidepressants on pain. Essentially, two mechanisms have been emphasized in the literature (Feinmann, 1985): (i) a direct analgesic effect on pain (ii) a mood-elevating or euphoriant effect (on depression) that in turn reduces pain.

Analgesic effects of antidepressants. Antidepressants have been recommended for pain at least since Paoli et al. (1960) reported that impiramine reduced the pain of several ailments. The few well-controlled experiments utilizing laboratory pain (e.g., Chapman, 1976) have failed to produce evidence of a direct analgesic affect of doxepin. However, there are clinical data that nondepressed patients do obtain relief from pain with imipramine (McDonald Scott, 1969; Gringas, 1976) or amitryptiline (Gomersall & Stuart, 1973) raising the possibility of a direct analgesic effect of certain tricyclic antidepressants. A survey of the records of 282 pain patients receiving antidepressants showed that 48% of patients attained marked improvement in pain from antidepressants of which amitryptiline was the most commonly used -- in 58% of the sample (Richeimer, Bajwa, Kahraman, Ransil & Warfield, 1997). In one of the better known studies using random assignment in a double-blind crossover design, Watson et al. (1982) found that amitryptiline was superior to placebo in relieving pain but this was independent of any change in depression. Nilsson & Knorring (1989) reviewed 42 studies of clomipramine for acute and chronic pain, and found pain reduction regardless of depressive symptoms, but the authors acknowledged the lack of proper assessment of depression in most of these studies. This implies a direct analgesic effect of antidepressants but it could also be due to the sedative or relaxant effects of antidepressants (Aronoff, Wagner & Spangler, 1986).

Not knowing the precise depression status of the pain patients, it is difficult to attribute the observed effect of antidepressant medication to analgesia alone. This is because of the reciprocal effects of pain and depression; a change in the latter can be responsible for a change in the former. Definitive evidence of the analgesic effect of antidepressants warrants demonstrations of pain relief in pain patients *without depression.* In a randomized, double-blind crossover study of amitryptiline on chronic pain patients without depression, Van Kempen, Zitman, Linssen and Edelbroek (1992) found that only 12 out of 34 patients achieved more than 50% reduction of their pain. Two patients attained between 25% and 50% pain relief but the majority obtained negligible or no pain relief. Van Houdenhove, Verstraden, Onghena & De Cuyper (1992) used an even more elaborate design to test the supposed analgesic effects of antidepressant medication. Within a double-blind placebo-controlled trial with mianserin, they compared four groups of patients: (a) nonorganic chronic pain plus depression, (b) organic pain plus depression, (c) organic pain without depression, or (d) depression alone. As much as 41% of patients dropped out because of severe side effects. Over the 12-week trial, no significant change in MPQ scores of pain was found in any of the three groups with chronic pain. This was despite a significant decline in BDI scores for depression. Even at the individual level of analysis, there was no evidence of pain reduction. The authors concluded that the antidepressant medication had no analgesic effect.

Also note that the physiological basis of pain is an arousal mechanism, whereas that for depression is quite the opposite: deactivation and a slowing down of functions. So, antidepressants, when they do produce pain relief, could be doing so by a mechanism other than analgesic medication.

Mood-elevating effects of antidepressants. Several studies have reported encouraging results for antidepressant use in headache (Lance & Curran, 1964; Couch et al. 1976; Noone, 1977), low back pain (Hameroff et al. 1982; Jenkins et al., 1976), rheumatic pain (Delle Chiaie & Teodori, 1985; MacNeill & Dick, 1976), post-herpetic neuralgia (Hanks, 1981; Taub, 1973; Taub & Collins, 1974) and heterogeneous pain syndromes (Blumer et al. 1980; Carosso et al., 1979; Clark, 1981; Duthie, 1976; Moore, 1980). As reviewed by Aronoff and Evans (1982), the response rates in these studies ranged from 44% to 70%, with an average of 62%, notwithstanding low dosages of the tricyclic antidepressants. However, depression can dissipate on its own. Kramlinger, Swanson and Maruta (1983) found that 90% of definitely depressed chronic pain patients showed resolution of their depression by the end of a 3-week inpatient pain management program during which none of the patients received antidepressants. The authors explained this largely with reference to cognitive change e.g., improved understanding of pain, acceptance of pain, and enthusiasm about returning home. Caution should also be exercised in view of many early antidepressant studies in this group not meeting one or more criteria for clinical trial research be it random assignment, double-blind procedure or placebo comparison.

The studies that did incorporate placebo groups (e.g., Evans et al., 1973; Jenkins et al. 1976; Lindsay & Wyckoff, 1981) generally reported no between-group differences although within-group changes were in the desired direction. This raises the possible role of motivation, attitude, expectation, and other nonspecific psychological variables governing antidepressant effects on pain. Patients who conceptualize their condition as treatable by (antidepressant) medication, have a strong will to get better and are self-efficacious about the outcome of medication, and hence likely to respond favorably to the effects of such medication. A recent aggregation of results from multiple studies strongly supports this reasoning. In their meta-analysis, Kirsch & Saperstein (1999) found that the average pretreatment-to-posttreatment change in depression among patients receiving antidepressant medication was 1.55, but the same dependent measure for placebo averaged an effect size of 1.16. As the authors inferred, "75% of the effect of antidepressant medication can be duplicated by administration of an inert placebo" (p. 505). In the context of pain too, it has been argued that antidepressants are not much more effective than placebo (Mendel et al. 1986).

The possible role of sedation and sleep cannot be ignored in any critical evaluation of antidepressants for pain relief. Sedation has been found to be the most common side effect of antidepressant medication in pain patients, reported in about 18% of patients (Richeimer, Bajwa, Kahraman, Ransil & Warfield, 1997). Drawing upon many years of clinical observations at the Boston Pain Center, Aronoff and Evans (1982) noted that doxepin administered at bedtime improved sleep well before improving mood (the latter taking anywhere from a week to three weeks). As patients wake up feeling more rested and relaxed, their pain becomes less bothersome and therefore it tends to be rated as having declined in intensity.

It is also important to note that the antidepressant dosage reported in most of the studies cited above was 50-100 mg per day. This is only about half the dose range of the same medication used for treating depression. Moreover, plasma levels of these drugs are far lower than the therapeutic levels observed in the treatment of primary depression. This may further support the intervening role of behavioral changes such as relaxation and sleep and attitudinal variables pertaining to medication and illness.

Side effects. The sedative effect of antidepressants does not come without cost. Antimuscarinic effects are common. Patients tend to complain of dry mouth, urinary retention, and CNS changes such as memory difficulties, confusion, and delirium. Even more hazardous are the cardiovascular effects, namely, orthostatic hypotension, increased heart rate, and hypertensive crises (when combined with foods containing large amounts of tyramine). These may be especially precarious in the elderly and chronically ill (Blackwell, 1987; Halper & Mann, 1988; Roose, Glassman, Siris et al. 1981). Of course, the different classes of antidepressants pose varying risks. MAOI's are associated with the tyramine effect and hypotension but are rarely prescribed anymore. TCA's are the most commonly used antidepressants for pain patients and are associated with heart rate increases and antimuscarinic effects. HCA's are associated with a bit of most side effects. By far, the SSRI's have the least side effects but are rarely used in pain patients (Merskey & Moulin, 1999).

Antidepressant dosage is always adjustable to minimize toxicity while boosting the desired effects. This is very much a trial-and-error exercise, although broad clinical guidelines exist (Richeimer, Bajwa, Kahraman, Ransil & Warfield, 1997; Stauffer, 1987). Paramount among these is the need to forewarn the patient of possible side effects and then start at a low dose -- typically about one-fourth of the recommended antidepressive dose. Typically, this is about 25mg (for TCA's) to be administered at bedtime. This may be increased in a stepwise fashion until the side effects, though present, are tolerable and outweighed by symptom relief. The patient should be consulted in the titration of the dose and the clinician should closely monitor the patient for overdose even though these drugs are generally not addictive. Desipramine or nortriptyiline are recommended for elderly or frail patients unable to tolerate antocholinergic side effects or sensitive to hypotension. Amitryptiline and doxepin are among the antidepressants prescribed for younger pain patients especially those with insomnia. The more intractable the depression, the more experimental the prescriptions tend to be. For instance, in the treatment of central pain and associated depression, Gonzales (1995) proposes a three-step process which is itself made up of several individual trials:

> *Step 1*…Agents that have been studied and should be used first are amitryptiline and, if anticholinergic side effects are problematic, nortryptiline. …anticonvulsants such as carbamazepine may also be efficacious, particularly if the pain has a lancinating, sharp, stabbing component… Phenytoin in doses of 300 mg/d or higher may also be administered. Nontryclic antidepressants, such as trazadone, have also been reported to be helpful.., Opioid analgesics can also be used, although high doses may be necessary… *Step 2*. When tricyclics, other antidepressants, and opioid analgesics are not efficacious, I add adrenergic agents, such as clonidine and β-blocking drugs, such as propanolol. I also use naloxone-containing agents – specifically, Talwin NX, which contains both pentazocine and naloxone. If the patient has been off opioid agonists or other mixed agonist-antagonist agents for at least 1 to 2 weeks, a trial with IV naloxone (0.4 to 2.0 mg over 5 minutes) can be given before starting the pantazocine-naloxone combination… Studies have reported good results with mexiletine, but I have not experienced this. Lidocaine infusions have not been successful in my patients, either…*Step 3*. Treatment options for refractory patients include dorsal root entry zone (DREZ) and spinal cord stimulation…
> (S15)

Some of the conflicting results in this area may be related to differences in type and severity of pain, and type and dosage of antidepressant drug administered -- as apparent in a tabulative review of the literature (France, Houpt, & Ellinwood, 1984). They could also be attributable to extraneous variables including degree of disability and participation in psychotherapy for depression. As noted by France et al. (1984), some studies are also difficult to interpret because of the combination of antidepressant medication with other drugs like phenothiazines, antiepileptic drugs, lithium, and pain killers. There is also a need to distinguish the effects of antidepressants in patients having depression secondary to pain from patients with depression that predates the pain, as well as the other interactive relationships between depression and pain discussed earlier. One of the few studies to consider this issue (Bradley, 1963) found that patients with concurrent onset of pain and depression obtained relief from both these conditions when administered antidepressants, whereas patients whose depression accompanied pain obtained relief only from depression when given antidepressants.

In summary, antidepressants do benefit pain patients. The primary efficacy of antidepressant medication in this population is in reducing depression rather than pain. There are relatively few well-controlled studies of pain relief among nondepressed patients. In reviewing these studies, Max (1994) found consistent analgesic effects only in the case of neuropathic pain. He also considered the possibility that some of these effects might have been mediated by the side effects of antidepressants. The idea of a direct analgesic effect is also weakened by the lack of corroborative data on neural or biochemical changes. This is partly a result of difficulties in collecting these kinds of data from humans already faced with the demands of participation in research on this issue. Animal studies are riddled with conflicting results too. Siegel et al. (1983) reported analgesic effects of TCA's that exceeded that of aspirin, nonreversible by naloxone but attenuated by reserpine which depletes CNS monoamines. However, Gonzales (1980) found minimal signs of anti-inflammatory activity in animals given antidepressants, and many other animal studies turned up short on evidence of analgesic activity during antidepressant medication (e.g., Botney & Fields, 1982; Leu & Wang, 1975; Spencer, 1976).

Morever, the same findings observed in humans may be attributable to the sedation and rest that occur much sooner than any discernible changes in depression or pain after antidepressant use. The changes in depression that follow later in time seem to occur at doses of antidepressants that are typically subtherapeutic when treating primary depression. This raises the further possibility of motivational, expectancy, and attitudinal factors influencing the response to this set of psychotropic drugs.

Among the other options for antidepressant medication are the monoamine oxidase inhibitors (e.g., Merskey & Hester, 1972) but these have been virtually abandoned for pain patients since the advent of the tricyclics. More recently, with the advent of fluoxetine (or Prozac) for the treatment of depression, selective serotonin reuptake inhibitors (including zimelidine) have attracted some interest. As pointed out by Merskey & Moulin (1999), this new class of antidepressants spares patients many of the side effects of the trcicylics; however, they are far less effective for pain patients and hence used infrequently.

Other problems/issues/questions. Some symptoms of depression may respond to medication whereas other depressive symptoms may not. Most studies use global scores that obfuscate such differential effects which could be related to different mechanisms. Also, there is a need to differentiate between clinical versus subclinical levels of depression or major depression versus dysthymia. To say that a patient was not depressed might mean that the patient's scores did not reach clinical significance, yet the low levels of depression might have responded to the antidepressant medication and thereby relieved pain.

There is a general lack of pharmacological specificity in psychotropic drugs. Antidepressants have found use as sedatives, mood-elevators, analgesics, and so on. Neuroleptics have found use in treating psychoses as well as depression. Claims have also been made of analgesics producing antidepressant effects.

Studies differ greatly in configuration and design. There is also a tendency to rely on the number counts of patients improved and of studies with significant effects. Better than that would be a meta-analysis of the literature so that effect sizes are generated for each study. This common metric permits meaningful comparisons across studies, and grouping of effect sizes according to methodological properties. A start in this direction has been made by Onghena and Van Houdenhove (1992). Their results, also evaluated by Max (1994), do suggest a moderate analgesic effect size of 0.55 for antidepressants, this being marginally higher in the few investigations of neuropathic pain or postherpetic pain.

There is a need to consider antidepressant effects within the context of each of the six primary interrelationships between pain and affect: affect as predisposing factor, as precipitant, as co-occurrent, as aggravator, as consequence, as perpetuating factor; and of course, affect can be independent of pain. There is also a reciprocal or cyclical relationship in which pain drives affect which in turn impacts on pain (this really represents a combination of two of the foregoing relationships). Antidepressants may alleviate both depression and pain when the depression precipitates or aggravates pain but less so when the depression is a consequence or co-occurrent of pain. Antidepressants are also likely to alleviate pain and depression when the pain is perpetuated by depressive events or the result of depressive traits. These hypotheses would be premised on the essential mood-altering function of these drugs. Disconfirmation of these hypotheses would suggest alternate functions and mechanisms for antidepressant drugs on pain sufferers.

Ironically, most of the studies in this area have been directed at determining the analgesic rather than antidepressant properties of TCA's in pain patients. This may be indicative of some sort of confirmatory bias on the part of those who view their main mission as one of *pain* management.

Integrated Treatment

Many studies have tackled the problem of depression within the framework of multidisciplinary pain management. Kramlinger, Swanson and Maruta (1983) ran an inpatient multidisciplinary treatment program for 100 patients with chronic pain (predominantly back pain) seen at the Mayo Clinic. Of these, 25 were definitely depressed, 39 were probably depressed, and 36 were not depressed, as defined by RDC criteria for major depression. The treatment program lasted three weeks and centered on self-management techniques, minimization of medication, and helping patients and their families cope with the pain. Although no significant differences emerged between the depressed versus nondepressed on the Hamilton Rating Scale, scores on this scale declined significantly between the time of admission and dismissal for all groups.

The foregoing success was replicated in another sample of 100 inpatients in the same multidisciplinary pain management program at the Mayo Clinic (Maruta, Vatterott & McHardy, 1989). A total of 54% of these patients showed either definite or probable depression according to RDC criteria. They underwent behavior modification, reduction of medication, biofeedback-assisted relaxation, education, participation of family members, group discussion, and supportive counseling. At the conclusion of the program three weeks later, 98% of the depressed patients were no longer depressed, and 85% of these remained depression-free at long-term follow-up approximately 12 months later.

The outcome of multidisciplinary pain management on depression is not site-specific and other centers have reported similar results. For example, a 4-week multidisciplinary pain management program (of 5 days per week) at the Center for Rehabilitation in Lake Forest Hospital, Illinois led to significantly reduced BDI scores in a sample of 94 patients (Burns, Johnson, Mahoney, Devine & Pawl, 1998). The program which encompassed physical and occupational therapy, individual and group CBT, biofeedback, education about pain, and treatment by a physician, produced an effect size of 0.58 which is indicative of moderate improvement.

Other variations of multidisciplinary pain management programs that also remediate depression have been outlined. For example, Verman and Gallagher (2000) proposed a 12-14 session program with a strong psychoeducational component, continuous assessment with the aid of diaries and dynamic charts, in addition to the standard interventions such as relaxation, biofeedback, and individual and group psychotherapy. Philips and Rachman (1996) have outlined a manual of multidisciplinary pain management with attention to depression, other mood disturbances and general functioning. It merits mention that such multidisciplinary efforts are not only efficacious but also cost-effective (Cipher, Fernandez, & Clifford, 2001).

Treatment Responsiveness and Prognosis

It has been a clinical observation for some time that pain patients who are depressed are more likely to drop out of treatment or relapse after treatment (Painter, Seres & Newman, 1980). Blanchard, Andrasik, Neff, Arena, Ahles, Jurish, Pallmeyer, Saunders, Teders, Barron, & Rodichok (1982) noted that depression in headache sufferers predicted poor response to biofeedback and relaxation treatments. However, a broader psychosocial rehabilitation program (Kramlinger, Swanson & Maruta, 1983) produced comparable treatment outcome for depressed and nondepressed pain patients.

In closely examining the responsiveness of depressed pain patients to rehabilitation, Kerns and Haythornthwaite (1988) incorporated psychometric scores as well as attrition rates within their outcome measures. With regard to the latter, 72% of depressed patients did not complete the treatment program as compared to 52% from a mildly depressed group and 51% from a nondepressed group. However, for those depressed patients who did complete treatment, no significant relation emerged between depression severity and psychometric measures of pain and life interference. There was a general improvement in all groups of completers between pre- and posttreatment.

Conclusion

Several scholars have noted the inconsistency of epidemiological data on prevalence of depression in the chronic pain population. Some have pointed to a 57% margin in prevalence estimates (Smith, 1992) while other lists show a 10-100% range in prevalence of depression in pain patients (Romano & Turner, 1977). In fact, the range is even wider. As low as 0% has been reported (Ehlert, Heim & Hellhammer, 1999) and as high as 100% has been reported (Violon, 1980).

How do we smooth out such epidemiological discrepancies? By separating the epidemiological statistics according to types of pain, greater consistency of results can be obtained as shown earlier. Any attempt to integrate the disparate epidemiological data must also take account of sample size. Perhaps one way of doing this is by weighting each prevalence statistic by sample size, as in the review of depression in back pain (Sullivan, Reesor, Mikail & Fisher, 1992). Finally, Banks and Kerns (1996) have shown that organizing studies according to depression measures also brings some order to the prevalence data.

Pincus and Williams (1999) have complained: "The preoccupation with reporting the prevalence of depression in populations with chronic pain, and the investigation of the causal path between the two are misguided, based as they are on the concepts of depression and pain as independent and homogenous syndromes, but also because they rely on inappropriate measurements" (p. 215). Indeed, there has been an abundance of epidemiological research focusing on the co-occurrence of pain and depression and a profusion of investigations into whether depression precedes or follows pain. However, as evident from the present review, the epidemiological research has extended beyond comorbidity statistics to information on many factors governing the distribution of depression in the pain population. Efforts are also underway to generate norms and cutoff scores for depression in the chronic pain population and incorporate new approaches to measurement. As shown earlier, it is also possible to infer more than simple cause and effect relationships between pain and type of depression. The multiple ways in which these two phenomena interact are now identified and evaluated empirically, so that a new model of pain and depression is manifestly possible.

CHAPTER 5

Anger and Pain

Definition and Conceptualization

As pointed out in Chapter 2, the same aversive situations that produce fear and sadness often produce anger. It is hardly surprising that pain, being a complex and unpleasant experience with a variety of implications and attributions, would be associated not only with anxiety and depression but also with anger. Yet, the relationship of anger to pain remains relatively unexplored. The present chapter begins with definitions of anger, hostility, and aggression, then uses the same format of Chapters 3 and 4 to elucidate the possible interactions between pain and anger. As before, epidemiological, assessment, and treatment issues will also be critically surveyed.

Anger: A Classical Definition

Searching for the logical structure implicit in common sense views of anger, Smedslund arrived at the following definition of anger: "a feeling involving a *belief* that a person one cares for has, intentionally or through neglect, been treated without respect, and a *want* to have that respect reestablished" (1992, p.30). The person one cares for is typically the self; to be treated without respect is to be treated discourteously, unjustly, or in any manner deemed offensive; to reestablish respect is to undo the effect of the wrongdoing. This, according to Smedslund, is a classical definition of the term anger that is also reflected in lay usage of the word.

Elaborating on the concept of anger, Averill (1982) states that "... anger may be defined as a *conflictive emotion* that, on the biological level, *is related to aggressive systems, and even more important, to the capacities for cooperative social living, symbolization, and reflective self-awareness*; that on the psychological level, *is aimed at the correction of some appraised wrong*; and that, on the sociocultural level, *functions to uphold accepted standards of conduct*" (p. 317).   This definition emphasizes the interpersonal conflict that is perceived or interpreted and the motivated behaviors that result from anger.

Psychological Perspectives on Anger

Nuances aside, most scholars of psychology converge on two main defining features of anger: cognitive appraisal and action tendency. These features may receive varying degrees of emphasis but they are viewed as common to all emotions.

Focusing on the cognitive structure of emotions, Ortony, Clore, and Collins (1988) propose that anger is a compound emotion linking an attribution about the action of an agent to an assertion about one's well being. Specifically, there is disapproval of someone else's blameworthy action (reproach) combined with being displeased about the related undesirable event (distress).

Frijda, on the other hand, focuses on the unique action tendencies associated with anger. These may be antagonistic or aggressive tendencies designed to restore control, seek redress, or remove obstruction (Frijda, 1986; Frijda, Kuipers & ter Schure, 1989).

Together, the *cognitive appraisal* and *action tendency* peculiar to the emotion of anger amount to a definition not unlike Smedslund's (1992) classical definition of anger in terms of belief and want. Like all emotions, anger can also be characterized along two quantitative dimensions, namely, valence and intensity. Anger is extremely negative on the valence dimension, meaning that it is an intrinsically unpleasant experience (notwithstanding its possible positive consequences).   As for intensity, anger varies on a continuum from a mild form known as annoyance to extremely high levels indicative of rage. What determines the intensity of this emotion are various appraisals about the situation, for example, the degree of judged blameworthiness, the deviations of the agent's actions from person/role-based expectations, and the degree to which the event is undesirable (Ortony et al., 1988). These appraisals are relevant to any attempt at understanding human anger, including that experienced by chronic pain sufferers. As shown later, the cognitive appraisals provide a platform for organizing the many attributions that chronic pain patients make about agents and their actions.

Related Concepts

Two terms related to the concept of anger are hostility and aggression. These need to be clarified so as to avoid the kind of confusion that arises from the interchangeability of these terms in common parlance.

Hostility is an attitudinal bias that predisposes the individual to view others as untrustworthy, undeserving, and immoral (Barefoot, 1992) and likely sources of provocation and mistreatment (Smith & Christensen, 1992). Not everyone may agree on the attributions of immorality, but there is consensus among psychological scholars that hostility is a dispositional variable. One who is hostile is not merely angry at a point in time but disposed/inclined to anger more often than not. Therefore, habitual anger is sometimes referred to as hostility (Buss, 1961; Siegel, 1986), even though the expression of anger in these cases may not be as intense or episodic. Hostility may thus be viewed as a trait or enduring proclivity, not to be confused with the emotional state of anger.

This brings us to the important distinction between state and trait anger. As defined by Spielberger, Jacobs, Russell, and Crane (1983), state anger is a transitory emotional episode, whereas trait anger pertains to a relatively stable pattern of personality attributes akin to hostility. Another dichotomy found in clinical discourse on anger is anger-in versus anger-out. As defined by Spielberger,

Krasner, & Solomon (1988), anger-in refers to the suppression of angry feelings whereas anger-out is aggressive behavior motivated by angry feelings. However, the outward expression of anger need not be aggressive, and verbal communication of anger also counts as anger-out. On the other hand, anger-in would entail neither aggression nor communication. Therefore, the terms "internalization" versus "externalization" have also been used as substitutes for anger-in and anger-out, respectively.

Mention should be made of a widely used term in clinical parlance: *passive aggressiveness.* As a mode of expression, this is probably intermediate between anger-in and anger-out. It involves the behavioral communication of anger in a covert manner typically involving noncooperation rather than overt aggression; thus it may take the form of procrastination, reticence, disengagement, and so forth. Passive aggressiveness is by its very nature less noticeable than overt/active aggressiveness but no less important as one of the anger-related facets of chronic pain. It was one of the personality disorders listed in DSM-III, discontinued in DSM-III-R, but returned in the appendix of DSM-IV as a disorder warranting further study.

Aggression is a behavioral reaction often involving various motoric responses in which the goal is to inflict damage (Bandura, 1977; Baron, 1977). Of special note here is that it is goal-oriented behavior. The relationship of aggression to anger is that aggression is the actualization of an action tendency often associated with angry feelings. As Averill (1982) reminds us, anger does not necessitate aggression but it would not be a stretch to argue that, more often than not, aggression implies anger. Aggression is a deliberate act of offending or inflicting harm on another. It can take the form of verbal offense or physical attacks.

Frustration refers to an objective set of circumstances that blocks an organism from its goal. This definition was adopted by social psychologists some time ago and it parts from common speech in which the words "frustration" and "anger" may be used synonymously. Put another way, frustration is not a subjective feeling in an individual but an objective state of affairs or a situation facing the individual. Just as facilitation is the promotion of access to a goal, frustration may best be viewed as a hindrance to a goal. Thus, one may frustrate the group process or facilitate it. Frustration from a goal frequently leads to aggressiveness (as demonstrated in early social psychological experiments), and this behavioral outcome is probably mediated by the emotion of anger. This is particularly so at an early stage of child development where means-ends discrepancies are at the root of most perceived anger (Fernandez, in press).

Unlike depression and anxiety, disorders of anger are unrepresented among the affective disorders of DSM. The only exception is "Intermittent Explosive Disorder" which is reserved for angry outbursts that are disproportionate to the provoking stimulus. Not classified as a mood disorder, Intermittent Explosive Disorder is grouped under the broad category of impulse control disorders like kleptomania, trichotillomania, and pathological gambling. The omission of anger diagnoses within mainstream psychiatric nosologies may be the reason for the lack of attention to anger as a clinical problem. Yet, anger does represent a disturbance of affect and like (its counterparts) sadness and fear, can certainly impair familial, occupational and other areas of functioning to the point of a disorder. Some scholars have therefore proposed labels for anger disorders such as generalized anger disorder and adjustment disorder with angry mood (Eckhardt & Deffenbacher, 1995). This mimics the existing classification of mood disorders. Alternative systems are possible as well. One approach is to differentiate those with intense angry episodes from those with persistent anger of a lesser magnitude, and from those with long-term unresolved anger – much like the variants of depressiveness. Yet, another system could be developed around anger expression styles, such as overtly aggressive anger and passive aggressive anger. The central argument here is that anger taken to a limit of frequency, duration, or intensity, is no less likely to impair functioning than is extreme sadness or fear; by virtue of that, anger warrants a set of diagnostic labels too.

Epidemiology

In view of the infancy of taxonomies for anger disorders, there has been little epidemiological data on anger, let alone data on the distribution of anger in pain patients. Averill's classic (1982) survey of 160 subjects (80 of whom were residents from the Greenfield area and surrounding communities in Massachusetts, and 80 of whom were introductory psychology students at the University of Massachusetts in Amherst), revealed that a majority (66%) reported anger between once and twice a week, and nearly half the subjects reported annoyance at least once a day. As he put it:

> Most persons become angry at least once a week, and nearly everyone at least once a month. (If relatively mild or easily forgotten incidents are counted, the incidence may jump to once a day). Many of these everyday incidents are by no means trivial or unimportant. In the present study the "most intense" incident within the prior week received a mean rating of about 7.0 on a 10-point scale, where 10 meant 'as angry as people ever become'. With regard to the experience of passivity, subjects generally reported being less in control of their thoughts and feelings than their behavior. The duration of the incidents, which was correlated with both intensity and the degree of behavioral inhibition, tended to be bimodal; that is, there were more incidents of relatively short (less than 10 minutes) and relatively long (one day or more) duration than there were of intermediate time periods (p. 165)

In pain research, anger is only just beginning to be included as an item in affective assessment. In the absence of diagnostic labels for anger disorders, investigators have relied primarily on anger scores instead of frequency or percentage of people with anger problems. Consequently, the data reported here generally do not relate to prevalence in the strict sense but to the mere presence of some degree of anger.

Presence of Anger in Chronic Illness

Stricken by illness, many individuals face persistent pain among other somatic complaints, limited feedback on etiology, and repeated treatment failures. These problems frustrate patients from their needs and goals, thus increasing the likelihood of angry reactions. Chronic pain syndromes are similar in this regard.

The chronicity of pain need not result in a constant angry presentation but the frustration that comes with pain may lead to different modes of anger expression directed inward and/or outward. Viney (1986), for instance, found that chronically-ill patients were more inclined to displace their anger indirectly than were those who were not chronically ill. These patients directed more anger towards others than did the terminally ill or the non-chronically ill subjects.

In those with rheumatoid arthritis, early studies had reported a notable presence of hostility (Cobb, 1959; Moldofsky & Chester, 1970). Surveying the personality characteristics of patients with rheumatoid arthritis, Achterberg-Lawlis (1982) concluded that anger is one of three dominant characteristics that include depressive symptoms and family/interpersonal disturbances.

Anger and hostility are also evident in recurrent illnesses such as genital herpes (Himell, 1981; Sacher, 1983). As Taylor (1987) pointed out, victims of this condition usually feel angry with themselves but also acknowledge the desire for retribution to others held responsible. There are also accounts of anger in conditions ranging from dysmenorrhea (Elliott & Harkins, 1992) to neoplastic disease (e.g., Jevne, 1990).

The inherence of angry feelings in chronic illness is poignantly illustrated in a case study of thalassemia (a chronic hereditary blood disease) by Georganda (1990). Apart from the commonly reported feelings of inadequacy and sadness, this patient evidenced resentment over the fact that she had to suffer whereas others did not. This was compounded by her reluctance to express anger for fear that she would be rejected.

Prevalence of Anger in Chronic Pain

Since anger arises in a range of chronic illnesses, it is not far-fetched to ask if it is a component of the chronic pain experience. One of the most extensive surveys undertaken on pain and distress confirms the presence of anger as well as its prominence in relation to other core negative affects. In a collaboration with the World Health Organization, Kristjansdottir (1997) randomly sampled 2400 schoolchildren aged 11-12 and 15-16 throughout Iceland. On a given day, these students were administered a 256-item questionnaire pertaining to pain, distress, attitudes and behaviors; this questionnaire which had been validated by experts was distributed in the classroom for anonymous completion. The response rate was 90.5 percent. As shown in Table 4, anger emerged as the most common concern affecting 76.5% of those with weekly back pain, 76.9% of those with weekly headache, and 78.3% of those with weekly stomach pain. This was followed by anxiety and sadness, respectively. The prevalence of anger increased with pain frequency and number of pains, so that among those with two pains per week, the anger rates went up to 63.6% for stomach and back pain, 84.9% for headache and stomach pain, and 87.0% for headache and back pain. For those with three pains per week, the anger prevalence rate was 85.7%. In all these cases, anger outstripped the other two components of the core of negative affect and all the other physical discomforts measured.

Table 4

Frequency of Anger Relative to Other Affective States Associated With Pain (Based on Kristjansdottir, 1997)

| | Weekly Affective Disturbance | | |
Pain	Anger	Anxiety	Sadness
Pain rare or never	39.8	15.8	10.9
Pain once a month	52.0	23.6	20.1
Pain twice a month	66.5	35.3	26.6
Pain once a week	54.1	27.7	21.8
Pain twice a week	80.6	58.8	43.8
Pain thrice a week	85.7	76.3	68.1
Weekly headache	76.9	53.1	48.5
Weekly stomach pain	78.3	60.4	52.0
Weekly back pain	76.5	50.4	49.1

One would expect that when a physical problem persists despite protracted diagnostic work up and repeated treatment efforts, it becomes extremely frustrating and therefore likely to evoke anger. Where is this anger directed at? Lumley, Torosian, Ketterer and Pickard (1997) report that the health care system is a target of much disapproval by pain patients. Fernandez and Turk (1995) have identified the following as common targets of anger in pain patients: the causal agent of the injury or illness, medical health professionals, attorneys and the legal system, insurance companies, employers, significant others, God, oneself, and (even) the whole world. Support for this list comes from a recent investigation by Okifuji, Turk and Curran (1999) of a sample of pain patients (mostly with low back or leg pain) referred to a multidisciplinary pain center. They found that about 60% of these patients were angry towards health care providers, about 20% towards attorneys, about 30% towards insurance companies, 26% towards employers, 39% towards significant others, but by far most pain patients (about 70%) were angry with themselves.

Angry feelings may be intensified in chronic pain syndromes when the origin of the pain is undetermined or when there is a suggestion that the pain reported is disproportionate to any objectively identified physical pathology. There may even be a suggestion, implicit or explicit, that patients are exaggerating their symptoms if not outright malingering. Few studies have examined this hypothesis in the chronic pain population even though the parallels with other chronic illnesses are hard to miss. What is available at this time are scanty bits of data and anecdotal reports about the co-occurrence of pain and anger.

For example, Schwartz, Slater, Birchler and Atkinson (1991) acknowledged the high frequency with which chronic pain patients exhibit anger and hostility in addition to depressive symptoms that are typically the focus of investigation. Similarly, Kinder and Curtiss (1988) have suggested that anger is a much neglected but important variable in the affective experience of chronic pain.

Empirical data from a study reported by Taylor, Lorentzen and Blank (1990) revealed that 61 chronic pain patients scored significantly higher than their spouses on the hostility subscale of the SCL-90. As explained earlier, a hostile disposition implies proneness to anger.

Schmidt and Wallace (1982) reported that one of the three factors emerging in a factor analysis of MMPI data from 50 patients hospitalized for low back pain was loaded with items from the Psychopathic Deviate, Paranoia, and Schizophrenia scales. The authors interpreted this as a sign of anger, hostility, alienation and reduced control among chronic pain patients.

The prevalence of anger in chronic pain patients may need to be qualified by gender differences. Sternbach, Wolf, Murphy and Akeson (1973) found males to be angrier than females based on scores on the psychopathy scale of the MMPI. MMPI data reported by Kinder, Curtiss and Kalichman (1986) also reveal a similar pattern. They suggest a greater role of anger in male chronic pain patients, whereas for female counterparts, anxiety was more prominent. A subsequent study (Curtiss, Kinder, Kalichman

& Spana, 1988) however, revealed a subgroup of both male and female chronic pain patients in whom anger played a unique role. In females, this subgroup was characterized by outwardly expressed anger, whereas in males the subgroup was characterized by suppressed anger. Burns, Johnson, Devine, Mahoney and Pawl (1998) found no interaction between gender and anger-in, anger-out, or trait anger in the prediction of pain treatment outcome. However, this is not to say that there were no differences between males and females to begin with.

Collectively, the reports cited above point to evidence of anger in many of the measures of hostility, sociopathy, and mistrust obtained from pain patients. That there is such a common denominator encourages the systematic use of more direct and specific measures of anger in this population.

Another important question to gauge the salience of anger in chronic pain is just how prominent anger is *relative to* other emotions. Most studies of emotional difficulties in this population report on depression and to a lesser extent, anxiety. However, clinical observations and the limited empirical data published on the subject indicate that anger is at least *as* prominent an emotion as sadness and fear in the experience of chronic pain.

Wade, Price, Hamer, Schwartz and Hart (1990) assessed depression, anxiety, anger, frustration and fear on visual analog scales (VAS) and regressed these on to VAS measures of pain-related unpleasantness and depression as indexed by the Beck Depression Inventory or BDI (Beck, 1978) and the MMPI. They found that when pain unpleasantness was at its minimum, it was significantly predicted by anger and anxiety and when the pain unpleasantness was at its maximum level, it was best predicted by anxiety. In addition, frustration turned out to be a significant predictor of all three levels of pain unpleasantness (minimum, usual, and maximum). These findings suggest the contributions of anger and frustration to the suffering of chronic pain. There is considerable overlap in meaning between frustration and anger however, the former typically being an antecedent of the latter (Feshbach, 1986). This may detract from the authors' conclusions about *unique* contributions of the VAS measures of emotion to the variance in pain and depression measures. Using the same VAS measures in the context of menstrual pain, Elliott and Harkins (1992) reported that frustration earned the highest mean score in a group of 130 undergraduate women.

Fernandez and Milburn (1994) assessed anger as a discrete emotion along with nine other emotions from a typology of Izard (1977) that included fear, sadness, guilt, shame, disgust, contempt, surprise, interest and joy. A separate VAS was used for each emotion. As expected, the group of emotions neutral or positive in valence (i.e., surprise, interest, and joy) was inversely related to pain-related affective distress. This contrasts with the negatively valenced emotions which are positively related (at a signficant level) to the affective component of pain. Furthermore, stepwise regression revealed that the subset comprising anger, fear, and sadness emerged as a significant predictor accounting for the largest portion of variance in the affective component of pain. These findings suggest that anger, fear and sadness form a triad of important negative emotions constituting the affective distress of chronic pain.

That the anger reported by chronic pain patients is indeed due to pain rather than extraneous factors is a question that had not been clearly answered. After all, pain sufferers may have various life circumstances that (independently of pain) frustrate and provoke anger. Therefore, Fernandez, Clark and Rudick-Davis (1999) attempted to partition the anger of pain patients into that which is attributable to pain and that not attributable to pain. A survey of 110 chronic pain patients voluntarily answered six questions pertaining to anger, fear, sadness, shame, guilt, and envy. Specifically, they rated how often they had experienced each of these emotions in the preceding 30 days. For each rating, they were also instructed to make an attribution of the degree to which each affect was due to pain using a 10-point rating scale. As in the previous research cited above, mean ratings showed anger to be the most dominant emotion, reportedly experienced by patients about

70% of the time; two-thirds of this anger was attributed to pain rather than extraneous factors.

The relative salience of anger in pain is also supported in an investigation of spinal cord injured patients. Summers, Rapoff, Varghese, Porter, and Palmer (1992) found that anger-hostility scores on the POMS explained 33% of the variance in pain severity. However, anxiety and depression as assessed by the Trait Anxiety form of the STAI and the BDI, respectively, did not add to the variance accounted for by anger. It must be pointed out that anxiety and depression are clinical syndromes encompassing a complex of psychological, neurovegetative, and physical symptoms; a more appropriate comparison with the emotion of anger would have been the discrete emotions of fear and sadness that are *subsumed* within these two syndromes, respectively. Furthermore, it is unclear why state anxiety was not chosen over trait anxiety as a predictor variable, since it is the transient rather than stable aspects of anxiety that are more likely to be related to pain.

The few studies of how dimensions of anger relate to chronic pain suggest that these patients are high on state anger rather than on trait anger. Feuerstein (1986) reported higher scores on ambulatory measures of anger in chronic low back pain patients as compared to asymptomatic controls. Gaskin, Greene, Robinson and Geisser (1992) assessed state anger by the State Trait Anger Expression Inventory (Spielberger, 1988), a successor of the Anger Expression Scale (AXS; Spielberger, Johnson, Russel & Crane, 1985). They found this variable to be an important predictor of the affective pain rating index on the MPQ.

Gender Differences in Anger Among Pain Patients

Unlike depression which is more commonly reported by females than males, anger is often thought to be more prevalent in males than females. This has been explained in terms of evolutionary theories about the functions of anger in hunting and territorial protection and the socialization that makes anger expression more acceptable in males than in females. Actual research on gender differences in this area is inconclusive. Some studies report no gender differences (e.g., Stoner & Spencer, 1987), others report more anger in males than females Fischer et al. 1993) and yet others point to significantly higher levels of generalized anger in females than males (e.g., Hashida & Mosche, 1988). For the pain population, there have been insufficient tests of this hypothesis of gender differences in anger. However, the few pertinent studies scattered over the literature are worth reviewing because of some light they shed on the issue.

Research by Kinder and colleagues provides some insight into gender differences in anger within the pain population. In the first of these studies, 42 male and 35 female chronic back pain patients were assessed (Kinder, Curtiss & Kalichman, 1986). Both the groups scored about 18 on trait anger (as measured by the State Trait Personality Inventory (STPI., Spielberger et al., 1979) differed a little more on state anger (males averaging 13.02, females averaging 11.46), and were nearly identical on measures of anger-in (about 14) and anger-out (14.5). In a subsequent study of 76 male and 68 female chronic low back pain patients (Kinder, Kalichman & Spana, 1988), mean scores were provided for each subscale of the MMPI as well as STPI and the AXS. On the Pd subscale of the MMPI which is closely related to anger, there were minimal gender differences whether the results were broken down by profile type or averaged across profile types; in the case of the latter, the mean scores were 62.55 and 63.97 for females and males, respectively. Similarly, mean scores for trait anger were highly convergent (18.93 for females, 19.15 for males), for state anger they were slightly higher for males (14.11) than females (12.86), for anger-in, 14.55 for males and 14.69 for females, and for anger-out, 15.23 for males and 14.76 for females. While these data provide valuable norms for interpreting scores, they echo the earlier lack of significant gender differences in anger among pain patients. Finally, in the study by Kinder, Curtiss and Kalichman (1992), anger scores for 52 male and 177 female headache patients were highly similar except for a "psychopathological" subgroup defined according to MMPI configurations. Only in this subgroup did females show notably higher scores on trait anger, state anger, anger expression, anger-out and lower scores on anger-in and anger control.

Further independent investigations have also confirmed the general absence of significant gender differences in anger among chronic pain patients. Using the Anger Expression Inventory, Tschannen et al. (1992) found slightly higher anger-in scores for males and slightly higher anger-out scores for females. Using the SCL-90, Taylor, Lorentzen and Blank (1990) found mean hostility scores of .96 and .93 for males and females respectively, thereby supporting the null hypothesis of no differences.

Burns, Johnson, Mahoney, Devine and Pawl (1996) assessed 54 females and 73 males suffering from chronic musculoskeletal pain and awaiting admission to a multidisciplinary pain treatment program. Among various measures were the Cook-Medley Hostility Scale, and the anger-out and anger-in subscales of the AXS. Men were slightly higher on hostility and anger-in while women were slightly higher on anger-out, but these differences were far from statistical significance.

Okifuji, Turk and Curran (1999) recently employed a version of the TRAPS (Fernandez, 1996) to identify the targets of anger in pain patients. In this test, patients rated the degree of their anger toward each of nine relevant targets in addition to their overall degree of anger. Given this, 65% of males and 71% of females from a sample of 96 chronic pain patients evidenced some level of anger. This difference, however, was not statistically significant. Males and females did not differ in their overall anger intensity nor did they differ in their ratings of anger toward individual targets.

In summary, no appreciable differences have emerged between male and female chronic pain patients on state or trait anger. Anger is as prevalent among female as male chronic pain patients. The bulk of the research reports higher anger-in scores for men and higher anger-out scores for women, though these differences are marginal. In a subgroup of pain patients with extreme psychopathology, females appear to have higher levels of anger but this finding awaits replication.

Denial of Angry Feelings

When those in pain do not report anger, the question must be raised as to whether they may be denying it because of social desirability considerations or coping needs. In comparison to other negative emotions such as fear and sadness, anger may be particularly prone to denial in view of the societal norms and religious teachings that discourage or even disallow one from harboring or expressing angry feelings. Such denial probably accounts for an underestimation of this emotion among pain sufferers.

Recognizing the difficulties in admission of anger, Corbishley, Hendrickson, Beutler, and Engle (1990) reported that even though chronic pain patients may present an image of themselves as even-tempered, responsible, harmless good citizens, 88% of a sample of such chronic pain patients endorsed angry statements in the course of focused experiential psychotherapy (a form of gestalt therapy designed to increase awareness and expression of negative affect). Considerable effort was needed to unravel anger because patients were inclined to withhold or deny it. Nevertheless, in contrast with nonpain patients, those suffering from chronic pain showed a smaller range of affect without any of the positive emotions reported by the former group. Apparently, chronic pain patients are inclined to inhibit expression of anger and this may be because of the perceived social undesirability of this emotion.

Franz, Paul, Bautz, Choroba, and Hildebrandt (1986) extracted three factors from MMPI data from low back pain, headache and pain-free subjects: lack of self-confidence, strange bodily sensations, and frankness. The last of these factors primarily consisted of masculinity/feminity items of the MMPI, and pertained to the willingness to acknowledge or express anger. The three factors were then used as variables in a discriminant analysis which revealed that both headache and low back pain patients were distinguishable from pain-free controls by their tendency to deny feelings of anger and aggressiveness.

Inhibited Expression of Anger

Whether one admits or denies having angry feelings, a second variable of importance is the degree to which anger is expressed. The ventilation or expression of anger (nothwithstanding its tension-relieving properties) is often unpleasant to others, and this outcome can be a source of remorse for oneself. Thus, individuals who recognize their anger may still be inclined to suppress the retaliatory action tendencies that naturally accompany this emotion. For example, Pilowsky and Spence (1976) found a 53% incidence of "bottled up anger" in patients with chronic intractable pain -- a figure significantly greater than the 33% of outpatient pain patients with such anger.

The discrepancy between experience and expression of anger is indexed by the anger-in subscale of the AXS. Utilizing this instrument, Kerns, Rosenberg, and Jacob (1994) found that the internalization of angry feelings accounted for a significant portion of the variance in measures of pain intensity, perceived interference, and reported frequency of pain behaviors. On the other hand, the expression of anger as measured by the anger-out subscale of the AXS was less strongly (though still significantly) related to measures of pain intensity and reported pain behaviors.

Using the AXS too, Tschannen, Duckro, Margolis, and Tomazic (1992) found higher mean levels of anger-in than anger-out in both male and female chronic headache sufferers. Path analysis revealed no significant relationships between these two forms of anger expression, suggesting that the anger characterizing the experience of chronic headache is largely suppressed. Patients with non-cardiac chest pain have also been found to register relatively high levels of anger-in (Tennant et al. 1994).

Comorbidity of Anger With Other Affective Types

The co-occurrence of anger with other affective disturbance such as depressiveness and anxiety is illustrated in the existence of such diagnostic labels as "adjustment disorder with mixed disturbance of emotions and conduct" (American Psychiatric Association, 2000). This particular diagnosis encapsulates criteria for depression, anxiety, as well as anger. This is justifiable because most situations generate a variety of cognitive appraisals. In the case of injury, the loss of function may produce sadness and depression, the prospect of re-injury may produce fear and anxiety, and the agent of the injury may elicit anger. The same situation, thus gives rise to mixed emotions because of the mixture of appraisals directed at that situation.

It should also be noted that anger may occur as a reaction to other types of affect. In the context of psychotherapy, Greenberg & Safran (1990) refer to primary versus secondary reactive emotions, the latter being a byproduct of the former. In an almost paradoxical way, contempt can thus become a reaction to inner shame, jealousy can be a reaction to underlying feelings of worthlessness, and anger can be a defense mechanism against anxiety.

Significance

Why is anger a matter of concern? Are there any deleterious effects of getting angry? Most people are aware of the destructive potential of anger as when it culminates in aggression. However, the damage done by anger is not confined to the targets of anger but also found in the host or person experiencing anger. The following sections reveal a range of adverse effects of anger with special reference to pain patients.

Inhibited Anger in the Etiology of Pain

In keeping with the psychoanalytic notion that strong unpleasant emotions can be converted into physical symptoms, it has been suggested that suppressed anger might contribute to reports of pain.   Using a hypothetical provocation to assess subjects' awareness and expression of anger, Braha and Catchlove (1986) found that chronic pain patients as well as patients under routine surgery had difficulty appropriately expressing anger.   However, the former group was less likely to acknowledge their anger or to label it, and less likely to achieve a resolution of their anger.   The authors suggest that pain patients internalize their anger and indirectly express it through pain.   As noted, there is a common perception that anger is socially undesirable and in some cases at least, pain may serve as a more legitimate complaint and a means for getting attention and succorance.   However, such an interpretation is suggestive of a factitious condition, the incidence of which is relatively small in the chronic pain population.

Hatch, Schoenfeld, Boutros, Seleshi, Moore and Cyr-Provost (1991) reported that a sample of individuals with tension headache (averaging five headache episodes per week for 8.5 years), showed proneness to resentment, suspicion, mistrust, and antagonism in their interpersonal relationships as measured by the MMPI Cook-Medley scales (Cook & Medley, 1954) and the STPI.   Compared to headache-free controls, they were aroused to anger more often but more likely to suppress these angry feelings.   The authors seem to suggest an etiologic role of anger and hostility in the production of headaches.   However, their data are correlational and may well imply that the frequent angry states are a reflection of the high rate of recurrence of headache episodes; similarly, hostility in this case may arise as a function of the prolonged history of high frequency headaches.

Kinder, Curtiss, and Kalichman (1986) reported that for male chronic pain patients, trait anger acted as a suppressor variable of elevations on the Hypochondriasis (Hs), and Hysteria (Hy) scales of the MMPI.   They took this as a sign that there may be a relationship between the repression or denial of anger and the degree of functional overlay as measured by the Hs and Hy scales.

A more concerted effort to test the hypothesis that anger inhibition might contribute to pain was performed by Kerns et al. (1994). One hundred and forty-two pain patients referred to an interdisciplinary rehabilitation program were administered the AXS along with measures of pain intensity, pain behavior, interference and activity. Anger-in turned out to be the best predictor of pain severity as well as pain behavior, accounting for 16% of the variance in the former and 13% of the variance in the latter. After depression, anger intensity added significantly to the variance in interference and in activity levels. As interpreted by the authors, the suppression of angry feelings by pain sufferers is likely to increase the amount of pain and disability they experience.

It must be pointed out, however, that the above studies have utilized correlational data. Obviously, this does not permit inferences about a causal link between anger inhibition and pain. Going beyond multiple regression techniques, Connant (1998) introduced structural equation modeling to test the hypothesis that anger inhibition leads to perceived pain. The same instruments were used to measure anger in and perceived pain as in the Kerns et al. (1994) study. However, results led to a rejection of the above hypothesis, the correlation between anger-in and perceived pain being nearly zero. This conflicting result may be due to sampling differences, the Connant study being on spinal cord injured patients where there is often significant disability that motivates the expression of anger.

Inhibited Anger in the Etiology of Depression

There has been a long-standing notion in psychodynamic theory that depression is anger turned inwards (Arieti & Bemporad, 1978; Freud, 1934; Friedman, 1970; Gershon, Cromer & Klerman, 1968). Rosenzweig (1976, 1978) refers to "intrapunitive" persons who do not express anger outwards but instead turn it upon themselves with self-blame, thus running the risk of depression.

It has been well documented that depression is a pervasive problem among chronic pain sufferers, but little research has appeared on the possible moderating/mediating effect of anger on depression among chronic pain patients.   Achterberg-Lawlis (1982) reported that anger was associated with depressive symptoms, although this may have been mediated by the high level of family and interpersonal difficulties also observed.

Wade et al. (1990) used multiple regression analsyes to discern the predictability of depression from anger. It was found that VAS measures of anger significantly predicted scores on the BDI and the depression scale of the MMPI. No attempt was made, however, to identify whether the anger in this case was suppressed anger or expressed anger.

The possibility of inhibited anger as a predictor of depression has been examined using path analyses (Tschannen et al. 1992). This involved interrelating scores on the anger-in and anger-out subscales of the AXS with scores on the BDI and the Pain Disability Index (Tait, Pollard, Margolis, Duckro & Krause, 1987). As mentioned earlier, both male and female chronic headache patients reported higher levels of anger-in than anger-out. The path analysis indicated that suppressed anger was significantly related to depression that in turn was directly related to perceived disability.   Anger-in accounted for 32% of the variance in depression that in turn explained 21% of the variance in perceived disability.   This may be interpreted in terms of the intrapunitive aspects of anger turned inward that arguably render an individual susceptible to depression.

Burns, Johnson, Mahoney, Devine and Pawl (1998) studied 101 patients in a multidisciplinary pain treatment program. All participants had benign musculoskeletal pain. Various measures (e.g., pain severity, anger, and depression) were obtained one week prior to the 5-day per week program and on the day of discharge from this program four weeks later. Among the important findings were the significant negative correlation between pre-treatment scores for anger-in and reductions in depression ($r = -0.33$). However, this finding was restricted to men, there being no significant contribution of anger to depression in women. In other words, the more these male patients suppressed anger, the less improvement in depression they exhibited. This does fit with the psychoanalytic view of depression as anger-turned inward.

A further hint of the contribution of anger-turned-inward to the depression of pain sufferers comes from research by Okifuji, Turk and Curran (1999). Using the TRAPS, they instructed patients to rate anger towards relevant targets such as health care providers, insurance companies, significant others and oneself. It was found that depression as measured by the BDI was significantly correlated with anger toward self ($r = 0.52$) and that was more than the correlations between BDI scores and other targets of anger. Whereas the background variables in the regression model only contributed to 4% of the variance in depression, self-directed anger added a significant 27%.

Consequences for Interpersonal Relations

The pervasive anger that chronic pain patients experience also translates into difficulties in interacting with spouses, other members of the family, friends, and health care providers. Schwartz et al. (1991) found that 28% of the spouses of chronic pain patients reported significant depression. This was found to be attributable to patients' pain, anger, and hostility, and spouses' level of marital dissatisfaction.

Hostile or anger-prone individuals often have fewer and less satisfactory social supports (Barefoot, Dahlstrom, & Williams, 1983; Hardy & Smith, 1988; Lane & Hobfoll, 1992). In addition, they report interpersonal conflict at work (Houston & Kelley, 1989; Smith, Pope, Sanders, Allred & O'Keefe, 1988). With regard to chronic pain patients who are angry and hostile, there is a strong likelihood that their suffering of physical disability is worsened by psychosocial conflict brought on or aggravated by anger and hostility.

A systematic study of the relationship between anger, interpersonal exchanges and adjustment to pain has been conducted in 135 married pain patients (Burns, Johnson, Mahoney, Devine and Pawl, 1996). Among the tests administered to patients before admission to a pain program were the Cook-Medley Hostility Scale, the AXS, and subscales of the WHYMPI. Regression analyses revealed that anger expression and hostility were related to the punishing responses from spouses. At least in men with high levels of anger expression, these punishing, critical responses significantly reduced adjustment to pain. Spousal solicitousness, however, was not significantly related to adjustment. These findings are consistent with other reports that anger externalized to caregivers may elicit antagonistic reactions from spouses and thereby compromise adjustment to pain.

Consequences of Angry States on Physical Health

The effect of emotions on physical well being has been extensively dealt with in psychosomatic medicine. Research in this domain has delivered compelling evidence of the link between negative emotional difficulties and medical ailments such as headaches, asthma, dermatological eruptions, hypertension and cardiovascular conditions (e.g., Cheren, 1989; Wittkower & Warnes, 1977). More recently, a special volume was devoted to the role of anger and hostility in health and illness (Friedman, 1992).

Since it seems that angry states (overt anger or inhibited anger) are a salient feature of chronic pain, this may carry implications for the physical well being of pain sufferers (Beutler et al. 1986). Diamond (1982) implicates anger and hostility in hypertension as well as coronary heart disease. Integrating evidence from personality and social psychological research, he discovered that at least a subset of hypertensives are chronically hostile, conflicted about anger expression and inclined to be overtly submissive but inwardly resentful. As indicated earlier, the inhibition of anger is a well documented feature of chronic pain syndrome. This raises the possibility that chronic pain sufferers who are hostile but internalize their anger may be prone to developing hypertension through neurogenically mediated pressor reactions. On the other hand, those who are emotionally undercontrolled and overly aggressive are, according to Diamond (1982), less prone to hypertension but they are not without risk; they become more prone to coronary heart disease. So the anger associated with chronic pain syndromes, unless appropriately expressed and regulated, has the potential of producing threats to cardiovascular health. Of course, this threat generally develops insidiously over the long term. It should be noted that in the short run too, acute episodes of anger have been implicated in numerous heart attacks.

Beutler, Engle, Oro'-Beutler, Daldrup and Meredith (1986) have reviewed research suggesting that stress-provoked changes in immunological responsivity may be a result of chronic pain and associated anger. The authors argue that the blocking of the anger and other forms of emotional distress coinciding with chronic stress or pain can deactivate the production of endogenous opioids and natural killer cells. Such a state of affairs reduces the body's defense against disease, pain, and depression.

Throughout this body of research, it is increasingly apparent that the inhibition of certain emotions may be particularly damaging to the physical well being of individuals. As suggested by the work of Pennebaker (1989, 1992), the active and effortful suppression of negative emotions increases ANS and CNS activity in the short run and over time undermines the natural cognitive processes that promote health thus culminating in sleep problems, elevated cortisol levels, and increased visits to the doctor. Anger, being a strong negative emotion, tends to be socially unwelcome, and therefore particularly susceptible to inhibition and such concomitant problems.

Consequences for Health Habits and Life Style

It must also be pointed out that apart from the physiological mechanisms by which problem anger produces illness, there may be a further mediating role played by health-related behaviors. According to this point of view, chronic pain sufferers may be inclined to develop the kinds of poor health habits that place them at risk for yet other illnesses and difficulties. This is exemplified below.

Leiker and Hailey (1988) for instance found that high scores on the Cook-Medley Hostility Scale were associated with poor health habits such as neglect of physical exercise and self-care, improper nutrition and driving under the influence of alcohol or drugs. The authors state that especially in the case of cynical hostility (already noted in chronic pain sufferers) where there is a complex of anger, resentment, and suspicion, the individuals may develop a "why bother?" attitude to health that may predispose them to what is called an unhealthy psychosocial risk profile. In addition, such individuals may be prone to certain forms of reckless behaviors that compromise well being.

The probability of specific health-compromising behaviors may increase with cynical hostility. As observed by Schweritz and Rugulies (1992): "hostility is related to a consumptive life-style, which includes, at least, food, marijuana, alcohol, and cigarettes" (1992, p.87). A high prevalence of such unhealthy habits partially explains why hostility has been repeatedly found to be associated with all-cause mortality: cigarette smoking contributes to cancer and cardiovascular disease, and alcohol consumption increases the risk of accidents and violent deaths.

In short, those in chronic pain who develop cynical hostility may be susceptible to a maladaptive lifestyle characterized by behavioral excesses and deficits. Anger is also known to undermine impulse control and increased risk-taking. These changes may be responsible for the additional health problems that afflict chronic pain patients.

Consequences for Pain Treatment Outcome

Anger can be a major complicating factor in the treatment of chronic pain patients especially if it is directed at those in the health care system. Data from Lumley, Torosian, Ketterer and Pickard (1997) do support the idea that pain patients have negative attitudes to health care costs and health care effectiveness. Anecdotal reports by clinicians also attest to the pervasive dissatisfaction with health care that sometimes assumes the form of outright anger. The ramifications for treatment are profound and far-reaching.

Any treatment (be it medical or psychological) requires mutual trust, acceptance, and co-operation between patient and therapist. To cite an example, health care providers may have as their objective a gradual reduction of medication. However, if the pain patient is cynical, mistrustful and hostile, then therapeutic alliance will be undermined and the tapering of medication will be less readily attainable. In chronic pain rehabilitation, the patient may even be required to serve as co-therapist with considerable responsibility to assume personal control in implementing coping strategies for pain. Angry feelings would pose a severe hindrance to such an objective. A new study by Cipher, Fernandez and Clifford (2002) employed path analysis to confirm that angry/aggressive styles in chronic pain patients were indeed associated with poor treatment compliance. This noncompliance was in turn associated with lack of improvement in functional capacity of the patients.

Angry pain patients are also potentially disruptive of the group process common to pain management programs. Angry outbursts can certainly detract from the course and pace of treatment. Where blatant retaliation is absent, there may still be noncooperation and passive aggressive behaviors that (through social modeling) have an adverse effect on the motivation and behavior of other patients. Pain management groups depend not only on the therapist's skill but also on the modeling of positive behaviors by participants in the group. Moreover, chronic pain is likely to be an enduring condition that will require long-term adherence to recommended lifestyle changes. High levels of angry feelings are likely to interfere with long-term compliance. These feelings need to become the subject matter of treatment.

Finally, anger if untreated, may give birth to a vicious cycle in which treatment fails, hence aggravating levels of frustration and anger. The patient is thus trapped in a self-perpetuating rut of failure and frustration. This may be one of the key reasons why patients who have not improved in previous pain programs are progressively poorer candidates for success in subsequent treatment programs.

Interactions

As in previous chapters, we now turn to the different types of interactions between affect (in this case anger) and pain. It will be noted that although all these interactions are meaningful hypotheses, data are not always available to put them to the test. The field of anger-pain research is only just attracting interest. In time, more studies will be cited to fill the current gaps in this area.

Anger as Correlate of Pain

Kerns et al. (1994) recruited 142 patients (mostly male) referred to a rehabilitation center for interdisciplinary treatment of pain. The pain disorders were primarily musculoskeletal in site. Measures of anger were obtained using the AXS. Pain intensity was assessed by the MPQ, pain behavior was assessed by the Pain Behavior Checklist (Kerns et al. 1991), and interference and activity were assessed by the WHYMPI. The results showed significant correlations, the highest of which was between anger-in and pain intensity (r = .41). Pain intensity was also correlated significantly with anger intensity (r = .30), with anger-out (r = .24), and with anger control (r = .18).   Pain behaviors correlated highly with anger-in (r = .36), with anger-out (.25) and with anger intensity (r = .18). Significant correlations also emerged between anger-in and interference (r = .29) and activity (r = -.21), and between anger intensity and interference (r = .38) and activity (r = .29). So, anger levels were associated with subjective pain report as well as pain behaviors.   The particular relationship between anger and interference is consistent with the earlier assertion that therapeutic alliance diminishes with anger.

A similar but smaller sample of male patients with musculoskeletal pain was assessed by Burns, Higdon, Mullen, Lansky and Wei (1999) using the Cook-Medley Hostility scale, the AXS and the pain severity subscale of the MPI. Hostility emerged virtually uncorrelated with pain severity (r = .06), pain duration (r = .03) and number of surgeries (r = .00); this may be attributable to the choice of the Cook-Medley which is at best a crude measure of cynical resentment rather than trait anger.   Anger-out was uncorrelated with pain duration and number of surgeries, but more correlated with pain severity (r = .17) at a level approaching significance. Correlations with anger-in were not reported. The correlation between anger-out and pain severity lies in the direction of that found by Kerns et al. (1994) and would probably have reached significance had the sample been as large.

A slightly different approach was taken by Okifuji, Turk and Curran (1999) when they adapted the TRAPS for assessing anger in almost one hundred chronic pain patients. It was found that the intensity of overall anger was significantly related to pain as measured by the MPI (r = 0.35); this approximates the result reported by Kerns et al. (1994).   Overall anger was also significantly related to disability (r = 0.26) and highly related to depression (r = 0.52).

Ambulatory monitoring of negative affect and pain over six days was the approach chosen by Rugh, Hatch, Moore, Cyr-Provost, Boutros and Pellegrino (1990) to examine the relationship between headache and various types of negative affect in a small group of dental hygiene students. They found that just as those with headache had significantly higher levels of pain than those without headache, they had higher levels of anger and core negative affect than those without headache, this difference being marginally significant. In the case of frustration, this difference was clearly significant. It is unclear how these terms were defined to the participants, but (as explained earlier) frustration is intimately linked to anger. The outcome of this study therefore supports the idea that anger co-occurs with headache.

Controlling for the non-painful symptoms of a disease that might also relate to negative affect, Glover, Dibble, Dodd & Miaskowski (1994) compared cancer patients with pain versus those without pain. They administered a short form of the Profile of Mood States (Schacham, 1983) to both groups of patients who also rated the intensity and duration of pain. Results revealed significantly greater affective distress (including anger) along with fatigue and confusion in the pain than the pain-free cancer patients. Anger and depression were the two affective states significantly correlated with pain at its worst, while anger and anxiety significantly correlated with pain at its least. The correlations between anger and these ratings of pain intensity were in the region of 0.20. However, anger was not significantly correlated with number of hours per day or days per week that patients experienced significant pain.

Anger Predisposing Pain

In the earlier-mentioned study by Burns et al. (1998b), about a hundred patients with chronic musculoskeletal pain were given the 16-item anger content scale of the MMPI-2 (Butcher, Graham, Williams & Ben-Porath, 1989) as a measure of trait anger. Results did not support a link between this measure of trait anger and changes in pain ($r = -0.05$) or other measures of functional capacity over the 4-week program.

When the more accepted trait anger scale of the STAXI was used to measure dispositional anger, a significant zero order correlation emerged with measures of perceived pain, r = .24 (Connant, 1998). Parameter estimates of a structural equation model of anger-pain relationships revealed a standardized regression coefficient of 0.39 between trait anger and perceived pain, which was statistically significant. This finding was obtained from a sample of 118 spinal cord injured patients all of whom were victims of an accident rather than disease or illness of insidious onset, and most of whom reported pain in multiple sites at or below the trunk. Since the self-reports of pain and anger were collected at the same point in time, it cannot be inferred that dispositional anger predisposed these patients to have pain. Furthermore, in the absence of state anger scores in this study, it is difficult to separate the contributions of situation versus disposition in the production of pain.

Anger Precipitating Pain

To show that anger precipitates pain would ideally require experimental designs in which the anger is manipulated. Alternatively, prospective designs can be used in which anger and pain are charted over time. No studies of the latter type appear in the literature but a couple of experiments support the idea that anger might trigger headache.

In one of the earliest examples of this kind, Marcussen and Wolf (1949) showed that being placed in anger-provoking situations triggered migraine attacks in patients. This has since been confirmed in a recent experiment on both migraine and tension-type headache (Martin & Teoh, 1999). In this study, 75 headache sufferers were divided into subgroups according to whether or not negative affect ordinarily played a role in their headaches. All headache sufferers then performed an anagram-solving task that was difficult and accompanied by failure feedback. This was designed to frustrate them thereby producing emotions such as anger. Such a manipulation of affect led to a greater increase in headache intensity among headache sufferers than control subjects who participated in a neutral task. Moreover, this increase in headache was regardless of whether or not participants normally attributed their headaches to negative affect. The effect was observed in patients with migraine as well as those with tension-type headache.

Anger Aggravating Pain

As in the chapters on anxiety and depression, the question can be posed about whether anger has an intensifying effect on pain. For instance, could the threshold of an individual's back pain be lowered by anger arising from conflict with one's employer or other non-pain related circumstances? This is analogous to the research (reviewed in Chapter 3) on arachnophobic anxiety and its effects on pain. Unfortunately, there is no research yet to explain the modulating effects of anger on pain sensitivity.

Anger Perpetuating Pain

The possibility that affective distress can be a source of secondary gain that reinforces pain behavior has already been considered in the context of depression. Just as depression might elicit helping responses from others, anger might elicit submissive responses from significant others. This is a positive outcome, and this contingency may maintain pain behaviors on the part of the angry pain patient. However, to date, no data have been presented to test this hypothesis.

Pain Causing Anger

Here, we are referring to the very sensation of pain as a trigger for anger. Some scholars (e.g., Berkowitz, 1990) assert that this aversive sensation is neurophysiologically hardwired to produce anger in the service of a "fight" response. This has not been systematically investigated in humans. In the meantime, indirect evidence might come from a demonstration that pain reduction leads to anger reduction.

Mechanisms

Appraisal Mechanisms

The foregoing studies report largely on standardized test measures of anger and related constructs.   There have been no serious attempts to explore the wealth of cognitions subserving these measures.   Yet, affect science has confirmed that cognitive appraisals underly emotions, and appraisal structures are now clearly specified for most discrete emotions (Lazarus, 1984; Ortony et al. 1988).

By interviewing pain patients and consulting pain clinicians, it has been possible to identify an array of cognitive appraisals associated with the emotion of anger in chronic pain patients. These can be organized into categories reflecting the cognitive structure of anger. Because anger involves negative consequences for the self attributed to the blameworthy actions of an agent, there are two groups of interrelated appraisals that are the focus of chronic pain sufferers: the agent who is the object of anger and the action of that agent or the attributed reason for the anger. The adverse consequence perceived to follow from the action is undesirable in all cases and is implicit in the description of the action.

Fernandez and Turk (1995) have specified 10 pairs of action-agent appraisals that underly the anger of chronic pain patients. Firstly, anyone who caused the painful injury becomes the principal target of the patient's anger. For example, pain due to a traffic injury of someone else's fault often leads to continued blame and anger toward the culprit. Recurrent pain may become a cue for recall of the activating incident and thus re-ignite anger toward the culpable agent. In the same way, anyone responsible for transmitting an illness with painful symptoms is likely to become the target of the victim's anger as long as the pain persists. In the course of providing health care, physicians, nurses, and other professionals also face anger from their pain patients. This is particularly so in the event that the pain goes undiagnosed or misdiagnosed and when treatment fails to "cure" the patient of his/her pain. As mentioned in the defintion section of this chapter, the degree of anger is governed by perceived deviations of the agent's actions from person/role-based expectations. This means that the pain patient may have such high expectations of medical science that when treatment outcome falls short of these expectations, anger is almost inevitable. People who have had acute pain successfully relieved by analgesics are often frustrated and angered by doctors dealing with chronic pain which by definition is refractory to conventional medical treatment. Psychologists and mental health professionals are therefore an integral part of multidisciplinary pain management teams. Unfortunately, patients are further taken aback if not affronted by a referral to a psychologist or psychiatrist. This is often taken as a message that the patient's pain is psychogenic or "all in the mind". When the pain and injury become the subject of litigation, the patient is often put through an adversarial process that generates even greater anger. Related to this is the anger directed at insurance companies and third parties issuing monetary payments to compensate a patient for pain. Such processes are likely to be conflictual and also long drawn-out and frustrating to the point of extreme anger. By their involvement in this process, employers also become the target of the pain sufferer's anger. This is compounded if the claimant loses employment or is forced to retrain or retire from the job as the case may be. Notwithstanding social security or disability benefits, the pain patient often experiences considerable anger and resentment when s/he loses gainful employment. The pain sufferer may also attribute blame and experience anger towards their own significant others. Again, this may be related to expectations that are discordant with reality. Family members and friends are expected to provide a degree of social support, but this may become unreasonable after a point in time.   Significant others may refuse to absorb the continued transfer of duties and chores from the pain sufferer.   This may be viewed as an abdication of interpersonal support and become the grounds for anger and retaliation on the part of the pain sufferer. Chronic intractable pain may also deteriorate into an existential crisis in which the patient is disaffected with himself/herself, with God, or even with the whole world.   As indicated in the definition of anger, the target of anger can be the self if it is also the agent responsible for the action.   Thus, the person who brings on one's own injury or illness is likely to turn anger against oneself.   The person who asks "Why me?" and interprets the painful condition as an ill-fated event, may turn anger towards God or a divine being. This can be generalized to anger at the whole world when the self is viewed as a helpless victim in a world full of more fortunate, unhelpful, or cruel beings who are resented.

Fernandez & Turk (1995) have diagrammatically represented the flow of events from pain and its associated cognitions to anger and its consequences.   Essentially, attributions of the kind described above lead to angry feelings that generate action tendencies toward specific behaviors.   The intensity of the anger is modulated by further cognitive variables such as degree of blameworthiness and extent of adverse consequences for the patient.   The action tendency itself may be overtly aggressive or else covert as in noncooperation, subversion, and other passive aggressive tendencies.   Inhibition or actualization of these tendencies both carry health risks -- cardiovascular deterioration, depression, and aggravated pain in the case of the former, and interpersonal conflict, adherence problems, and certain behavioral excesses in the case of the latter.

Centrally Hardwired Anger

Although cognitions are integral to emotions (Lazarus, 1984), the possibility has been raised that anger is one of those emotions occasionally unmediated by thinking. For example, Tomkins (1991) speaks of free-floating anger as occurring independently of appraisals. But free-floating anger, like free-floating anxiety is a mood disturbance. As pointed out in Chapter 1, moods, unlike emotions, are more enduring than episodic, and not readily attributable to specific cognitive antecedents especially when they occur below a level of awareness or insight.

Yet, dysfunctional moods and emotions are often the targets of psychotherapeutic intervention. Rational-emotive therapy and cognitive therapy are premised on the assumption that emotional aberrations arise from distorted appraisals in need of correction. Insight-oriented therapies may attempt to unravel deep-seated beliefs and ideas originally accessible to the subject's consciousness. This suggests that the inability to report cognitive appraisals responsible for mood disturbance does not imply an absence of such appraisals since psychotherapeutic strategies often uncover latent cognitions that are not manifest to the subject.

The so-called cognitive-neoassociationistic assertion of Berkowitz (1990) is that certain stimuli like pain, foul odors, and high temperatures can (innately) trigger angry reactions without cognitive mediation. Challenging the cognitivist position on anger, Berkowitz and Heimer (1989) reported that even in the absence of reasonable blame, unpleasant tobacco smoke produces angry/aggressive reactions in human subjects. Similarly, inclement weather, accidentally stubbing one's toe, or the sound of another person snoring, can arguably lead to expressions of anger. The reason, according to Berkowitz, is that these are physiologically offensive rather than because we ascribe any psychological significance to them.

According to Izard (1993), the mechanism of anger in these instances may be subcortical. Le Doux (1987) has for instance identified a subcortical pathway by which pain receptors transmit afferent signals to the thalamus and on to the amygdala that releases responses such as anger. It is not coincidental that brain sites such as the amygdala and hippocampus that are physiologically linked to pain and aversion are really part of a larger rostral-caudal network subserving emotions (Heath, 1986).

However, one must be cautious in ruling out the mediating influences of cognition -- since information processing involves many steps from the most rudimentary such as attention and anticipation to memory and complex judgments; these may occur extremely rapidly and often below the threshold of detection (Lazarus, 1984; Lazarus, 1991). Besides, thought sequences can develop an automaticity that may elude one's awareness. The rapid conjunction of anger with aversive stimuli like pain may hence involve varying degrees and levels of cognitive mediation.

Anger and the Peripheral Nervous System

Anger is arguably associated with more physiological activation than is any other emotion. In their recent meta-analysis of almost 20 studies dealing with physiological patterning of emotions, Cacioppo, Bernston, Klein and Poehlmann (1997) found convergent evidence of increased diastolic blood pressure, skin conductance, stroke volume, cardiac output, peripheral resistance, finger pulse, and heart rate during anger. This is suggestive of an overall sympathetic nervous system activation. Such increases in arousal represent a form of stress that is likely to add to pain.

The symptom specificity model of Flor and colleagues (Flor et al. 1992; Flor & Turk, 1989) that has been invoked to explain stress effects on pain may also help illuminate a link between anger and pain. This model asserts that in some patients with musculoskeletal pain, there are signs of stress-induced tension at the site of pain or injury. For example, chronic low back pain patients have a tendency to higher electromyographic activity in the lower paraspinal muscles when compared to normals or patients with pain in other sites. These same back pain patients do not differ significantly from normals on EMG levels distal to the lower back or on measures of autonomic activity such as heart rate and skin conductance. This has been corroborated by Burns,

Wiegner, Derleth, Kiselica and Pawl (1997) who found that the pain reports of chronic back pain patients were positively related to stress-induced increases in lower paraspinal EMG levels but not to EMG changes in the trapezius muscles or to cardiovascular reactivity.

Adopting this line of reasoning, Burns (1997) set out to show that anger exerts its effects on back pain by way of increases in paraspinal EMG. Data from 102 chronic back pain patients in the Burns et al. (1997) study were re-analyzed to see if anger as measured by the AXS and hostility as measured by the Cook-Medley Hostility Scale were related to pain via changes in EMG or cardiovascular measures. Results revealed that while paraspinal tension increased during the stress of an arithmetic task, it did also increase during an anger recall procedure. Those high on hostility and anger suppression showed elevated paraspinal reactivity during the anger recall, while those low on anger suppression and hostility showed the reverse. No comparable changes were found in EMG of the trapezius muscle. As the authors concluded, site-specific changes in muscle tension may occur in chronic pain patients as a result of anger. These changes may not cause the pain but they seem to intensify it. In the case of headache, Martin and Teoh (1999) found evidence of changes in vascular variables (temporal pulse amplitude, R wave to pulse interval, and interbeat interval) during an angry/stressful induction that led to increased headache. This was interpreted as a sign of sympathetic nervous system mediation between anger and the pain of headache. In short, this gathers support for the mechanism linking anger to peripheral nervous system activity.

Assessment of Anger and Hostility

Approaches to anger assessment range from projective tests to physiological measures. The focus here will be on self-report questionnaires for assessing anger, hostility, and related constructs. The objective will be to briefly review these instruments from a user's perspective with special attention to aspects of importance to pain. In addition, suggestions will be offered for the assessment of specific targets and themes of anger and hostility in the chronic pain population. The reader is referred to Biaggio (1980), Spielberger, Jacobs, Russell and Crane (1983), Biaggio and Maiuro (1985), and Barefoot (1992) for reviews containing more psychometric detail on several self-report assessment tools for hostility and/or anger.

Buss-Durkee Hostility Inventory (BDHI). Developed by Buss and Durkee (1957), this is the most widely used self-report measure of hostility. Its two underlying factors are neurotic aspects of hostility as measured on two subscales (suspicion and resentment) and behavioral-expressive aspects of hostility as measured on five subscales (assault, indirect hostility, verbal hostility, negativism and irritability). There appear to be no published studies of the BDHI applied to chronic pain patients. The distinction between hostile outlook and hostile presentation would be relevant to many patient groups, but of particular value in the characterization of pain patients is the differentiation among various forms of hostile expression ranging from the passive to the active. It must be noted, however, that BDHI scores are influenced by social desirability. In other words, they probably yield an underestimation of hostility levels.

Overcontrolled-Hostility Scale (O-H Scale). The O-H scale of Megargee, Cook and Mendelsohn (1967) assesses the tendency towards rigid overcontrol of aggressive impulses culminating in occasionally intense outbursts of aggression. This may be particularly relevant to the unassertive pain patient who is reluctant to express anger or other conflicts because of its presumed social undesirability and/or psychodiagnostic implications. It is important to note that the O-H Scale was developed exclusively and largely studied in male subjects. Any attempt to apply it to overcontrolled hostility in a chronic pain population must consider this demographic constraint.

Hostility and Direction of Hostility Questionnaire (HDHQ). Unlike the O-H Scale which assesses impunitiveness, the HDHQ (Caine, Foulds, & Hope, 1967) assesses intropunitiveness as well as extrapunitiveness. The former factor includes subscales of delusional guilt and self-criticism, while the latter includes delusional hostility, criticism of others and hostile acting out. This is analogous to the anger-in, anger-out distinction. It is an important distinction to make since, as explained earlier, intropunitiveness has been implicated in depression, while the externalization of hostile impulses often leads to interpersonal conflict. Items on the HDHQ can be easily culled from the MMPI. Since many pain clinics have been routinely administering the MMPI, this makes it convenient to obtain information on the direction of hostility. By the same token, the HDHQ should not be used outside the context of the MMPI, as many of its items refer to pathognomic qualities (e.g., paranoia) and are hence susceptible to social desirability effects. In the context of the MMPI however, they can be interpreted with reference to the validity scales.

Cook-Medley Hostility Scale (Ho Scale). Also derived from the MMPI, the Cook-Medley Hostility Scale (Cook & Medley, 1954) is much more commonly used than the HDHQ. It assesses the cognitive components of hostility, in particular, such attitudinal variables as resentment and suspiciousness. Therefore, the construct in question is referred to as cynical hostility. This scale has been widely used in predicting certain cardiovascular health risks. There is also a study of chronic headache patients (Schoenfeld, Boutros, Seleshi, Moore & Cyr-Provost, 1991) that has uncovered high levels of resentment, suspicion, mistrust, and antagonism using the Ho Scale. One must be mindful, however, that the Ho Scale was actually developed to identify teachers with difficulty relating to their students, and later found to (surrendipitously) predict coronary artery disease. Its applicability to the chronic pain population would be convenient inasmuch as the MMPI has been a routine part of the clinical assessment of many pain patients. However, there is insufficient published research to support the unqualified use of this scale as a measure of hostility in pain patients.

Anger Self-Report (ASR). The ASR (Zelin, Adler & Myerson, 1972) utilizes several items from other anger/hostility assessment instruments to distinguish between the awareness of anger and the expression of anger. A total expression score is derived as a function of what the authors term physical expression, verbal expression, and general expression. In addition to such ways of externalizing anger, there are subscales for assessing intropunitive feelings like guilt and condemnation of anger. Many of the subscale scores correlate with those on the BDHI and (like the latter) tend to be influenced by social desirability.

Reaction Inventory (RI). The RI (Evans & Strangeland, 1971) uses hypothetical scenarios to determine potential anger-provoking stimuli. These can be organized into 10 factors: minor chance annoyances, destructive people, unwarranted delays, inconsiderate people, self-opinionated people, frustration at work, criticism, major chance annoyances, people being personal, and authority. The overriding construct being assessed is one's propensity to anger arousal. Since this refers to dispositional aspects of anger, it is not surprising that it correlates with scores on the BDHI.

Anger Inventory (AI). Almost identical in format to the RI, the AI (Novaco, 1974) aims to assess anger arousability in response to a variety of hypothetical provocations. Like the RI, it is also correlated with scores on the BDHI, and slightly correlated with social desirability scores.

Multidimensional Anger Inventory (MAI).   In more recent times, Siegal (1986) developed the MAI that is quite brief but more comprehensive than its forerunners described above. It assesses a range of anger-eliciting situations, and goes further to assess the frequency, intensity, and duration of anger by items that load on a factor called anger arousal. In addition, it assesses hostile outlook, and makes a distinction between two modes of expression of anger: anger-in and anger-out. Although it was designed primarily with cardiovascular patients in mind, its factor structure has been replicated in two populations that differ in age, geographic location, gender composition, and lifestyle.

State-Trait Anger Expression Inventory (STAXI).   Calling attention to the complexity of anger and its related constructs, Spielberger and his colleagues developed the STAXI (Spielberger, 1988). This represents an integration of two precursors, the State-Trait Anger Scale or STAS (Spielberger, Jacobs, Russell & Crane, 1983) and the Anger Expression Scale (Spielberger, Johnson, Russell, Crane, Jacobs & Worden, 1985).   Recently, it was upgraded to the STAXI-2 (Spielberger, 1999). What is unique about the STAXI is its attempt to assess angry actions alongside dispositional aspects of anger (i.e., hostility) as well as incorporate the assessment of modes of anger expression (anger-in versus anger-out) in addition to the ability to control anger. This not only makes it the most thorough instrument of its kind but it also allows the integration of diagnostic and prognostic impressions and treatment ideas from the administration of a single test. A case formulation can be made of whether the anger of a chronic pain patient is primarily related to frustration and perceived maltreatment (state anger) or else a sign of (premorbid) anger-proneness (trait anger). Overt expression of anger (anger-out) may be minimal but anger may still be experienced if anger-in scores are high. Thus, the individual's control of anger can range between overcontrol and undercontrol and thereby serve as a guide for treatment planning.

However, the operationalization of state versus trait anger by asking subjects to report how they feel "right now" and "how they feel generally" is somewhat misleading. As pointed out in Chapter 1, saying that I am angry right now could mean that the anger began two minutes ago or that it has been around for two days. On the other hand, saying that I am generally angry is also ambiguous since it could suggest that my anger is unremitting or that my anger is frequent. Another problem is that patients may be puzzled by the repetitive nature of many of the test items. Some of them may retort that they fail to see the purpose of being asked to respond to such similar sounding statements as "I feel furious", "I feel angry", "I am mad" etc.

Psychometrically, the factor structure of the STAXI as recently uncovered by Fuqua, Leonard, Masters, Smith, Campbell and Fischer (1991) has by and large confirmed the construct validity of this instrument. High coefficients of reliability and internal consistency are also reported for the STAS and AXS segments of the STAXI (Spielberger & Sydeman, 1993). Moreover, concurrent validity has been demonstrated by correlations between the STAXI trait anger and hostility measures such as the BDHI, while discriminant validity has been reflected in the negative correlations between anger-out and anger-in and between anger-out and anger control. Data are not available on the relationship between the STAXI and tests of social desirablity, but there are some indications that test-taking attitudes influence results. For example, Spielberger and Sydeman (1993) found that small negative correlations emerged between Trait Anger and the Lie Scale of the Eysenck Personality Questionnaire (Eysenck & Eysenck, 1975).

The Targets and Reasons for Anger in Pain Sufferers (TRAPS). The STAXI-2 is by far the most psychometrically sound and comprehensive assessment tool for anger and hostility. However, it was not designed for chronic pain patients per sé and therefore it would only be able to identify the broad dynamics of anger such as expression and control.

What is equally if not more warranted is information on the specific *targets* and *reasons* for anger experienced by pain sufferers. Clinicians who have to deal with angry and/or hostile pain patients would find it useful to figure out whom the anger is primarily directed at, and why that is so, in order to formulate an appropriate strategy to reduce this anger and its impact on the pain. Such information would, for instance, invite the use of cognitive techniques that can reinterpret the pain-anger relationship and replace maladaptive appraisals with more adaptive alternatives.

The 10 common objects of anger in pain sufferers and a set of 10 corresponding reasons have been organized into a form called the Targets and Reasons for Anger in Pain Sufferers (TRAPS) developed by Fernandez (1996). On one side of the form, subjects are asked to rate on visual analogue scales how much anger they feel towards each of the objects of their anger. On the opposite side of the form, they are instructed to identify the reasons for their anger and rank them in order of importance. (Note that the ordinal rankings can be substituted with nominal rankings or with interval rankings according to the intellectual-cognitive capacity of the subject and statistical requirements). The data thus derived would illuminate the relative importance of specific targets and reasons for anger experienced by those in chronic pain. The form is designed to be completed by clinicians on behalf of pain sufferers. This usually entails a 10-minute structured interview. For convenience, the TRAPS has also been adapted into a self-administered version (Okifuji, Turk & Curran, 1999).

Behavioral Observations

Barefoot (1992) has developed a scheme for coding angry behavior within the context of an interview. Known as the Interpersonal Hostility Assessment Technique, it codes four types of behaviors: hostile evasions, indirect challenges, direct challenges, and irritation. Averaging across questions in each category yields a hostile behavior index. This system has been used primarily in cardiac settings but might be an option for assessing anger in pain patients too. However, as Barefoot himself acknowledges, the interview is time-consuming, and requires considerable training on the part of interviewers. The inter-judge reliability of interviewers is also not as high as in most standardized psychometric tests of anger. Finally, the IHAT is not invulnerable to social desirability factors. Given that the interview represents a controlled setting, participants too may be in better control of their emotions than they would be in naturalistic settings.

Self-Monitoring

A time-honored technique for assessing anger in naturalistic settings is self-monitoring. This involves training the subject or patient to observe and record anger wherever and whenever it might occur in the individual's natural environment. Beck & Fernandez (1998a) and Fernandez & Beck (2001) have devised pocket-sized cards for this purpose. These cards may come with graphs with time and intensity axes for recording instances of anger. In this way, it is possible to get measures of the frequency, duration, and intensity of anger as it transpires in the natural environment. This method also minimizes the limitations posed by retrospective self-report on questionnaires.

An Integrated Assessment Approach

There is considerable overlap among the instruments for assessing anger and hostility. Yet, it is clear that some instruments outperform others in terms of comprehensiveness and psychometric qualities. The STAXI, in particular, stands out as the least dated and most promising instrument in this area. It is the instrument of choice for the assessment of anger and hostility.

Apart from characterizing anger in terms of the state-trait distinction, anger-in versus anger-out, and the control of anger, it is also essential to identify who the individual's anger is directed at and why this is so. To accomplish this, a form called the TRAPS permits a convenient way for patients to identify and rate the targets and reasons for their anger, thus demystifying this complex emotional experience. Moreover, the TRAPS is specifically designed with pain patients in mind.

As the STAXI and the TRAPS do not have built-in items for assessing test-taking attitudes, the Marlowe-Crowne Scale (Crowne & Marlowe, 1960) might be administered too. This would provide specific information on the extent to which subjects' responses are governed by considerations of social desirability. This is especially important since the expression or even experience of anger is widely viewed as unacceptable.

The integration of these three instruments together with self-monitoring methods allows breadth as well as depth in the assessment of anger and hostility in the chronic pain population. It is hoped that through further integration of this information with data on other negative emotions associated with pain, a more holistic picture will be obtained about the affective status of the pain sufferer.

Measurement Issues

Among the main difficulties in measuring emotions is the lack of psychophysiological specificity; this makes it questionable to operationalize emotions solely on the basis of such measures as blood pressure, heart rate, and finger temperature. Self-report measures are also needed to round off the picture. However, one particularly serious problem facing self-report measures of anger is social desirability bias. Unlike depression and anxiety which tend to be the subject of more open disclosure, anger is prone to concealment and denial. Social norms (themselves reinforced by religious proscriptions) discourage anger expression. As a result, the various "transparent" items on psychological tests of anger are often answered in a manner indicating social appropriateness rather than anger.   The extent of this problem can be quantified by administering separate tests of social desirability e.g., the Marlowe-Crowne Social Desirability Scale.   Scores on these can then be used to validate or invalidate scores on anger tests or else to introduce a correction factor.

Treatment of Anger in Pain Sufferers

Psychological Treatment

Cognitive Reappraisal.   Since anger, by definition, embodies appraisals of wrongdoing, one obvious approach to reducing anger is through reappraisal.   As in the reappraisal of depressive ideation, this entails disputing automatic thoughts and restructuring basic cognitive schemas that govern such thoughts. Some standard reappraisals involve reconsidering the intentionality of the wrongdoer, reevaluating the severity of the wrong, or finding some redeeming feature in the situation.   Thus, the chronic pain patient who is angry towards health professionals because of treatment failures, may be engaged in a dialogue that leads to a new set of countercognitions: "the doctor tried his/her best and is therefore not culpable", "the pain, though not improved, is no worse", and "the failure of one treatment modality does not exclude the possibility of successes by other means".

This kind of approach to altering cognitions by rational disputation, counter-evidence, or replacement with coping statements has been found to be successful in the regulation of anger (e.g., Deffenbacher, Dahlen, Lynch, Morris, & Gowensmith, 2000).   However, it is yet to be applied to the anger of pain patients.

Behavior Modification.   Keefe, Beaupre and Gil (1996) have offered some behavioral approaches to reducing the expression of anger in group therapy.   These include interrupting the discussion of anger with relaxation exercises, postponing discussion of anger, time-out procedures and the like. This may be appropriate when anger is clearly fueled by secondary gain. However, it also runs the risk of ignoring the critical difference between anger expression and anger experience. Inattention and interruption of anger may (temporarily) reduce the communication but not the experience of anger. Besides, frustration leads to anger and its concomitants, and frustration from the need to express anger is likely to make patients angrier; as they get angrier, the need for expression of anger increases, and thus the individual is trapped in a vicious cycle of escalating anger.

Other behavioral techniques such as behavioral contracts, stimulus control, and behavioral rehearsal might provide alternative avenues to the regulation of anger. These techniques have been parceled together as part of a preventive approach to anger (Fernandez, 1999, 2001). Although especially suited to children who (because of developmental limits) are less likely to respond to abstract cognitive approaches (Fernandez, in press), the behavioral prevention of anger is also worthy of application to chronic pain patients. The pain itself is unavoidable, so stimulus control would be contraindicated. However, because it is expected to recur, the pain can be something one prepares for. First of all, a contract against anger can be signed to get patients to agree ahead of time that they will not get angry even when the pain strikes. Such a commitment in advance may not abolish anger but reduces the likelihood of it occurring. Then, behavioral rehearsal can be used to equip patients with anger-regulation techniques such as relaxation when pain strikes and anger follows. The actual techniques may vary, but the rehearsal itself involves behavioral modeling and role-played behaviors.

Affective Remediation. Just as grief may last well beyond the point of loss, anger may linger for a long time after the provocation. The pain sufferer, for example, may develop a long-term anger (albeit at lower levels of intensity) following an injury and treatment failure that is long past. This form of residual anger is probably not suited to the preventive and interventive techniques mentioned above. Instead, it calls out for a method of last resort -- a method that relieves leftover anger using so-called experiential techniques. Unlike behavioral and cognitive counterparts, these experiential techniques are emotionally evocative. Hence, they may be simply termed affective remediation (Fernandez, 1999; 2001).

Affective remediation techniques abound in Gestalt therapy. One example is the empty chair technique which is ideal for expressing anger toward an individual who is beyond communication from the patient due to distance, death, or some other hindrance. Outlets may also be found in vocal or written disclosure where the recipient merely listens or attends to the disclosure without interpreting or offering recommendations. Expressive art may also be explored as a medium for the sublimation of anger. Though yet to come under serious scientific inquiry, these affective techniques occupy a meaningful place in the spectrum of anger regulation and clinically they are used more widely than is reflected in the published literature. Preliminary findings suggest that these techniques exert an additive effect on the benefits produced by behavioral and cognitive procedures (Fernandez & Scott, 2001). It is therefore recommended that this approach be adopted as part of a final phase in the regulation of anger in pain sufferers.

Integrated Treatment

CBT packages.   Because of their common origin in learning theory, cognitive and behavioral techniques have been customarily combined in the effort to treat emotional disorders such as anger. In fact cognitive-behavioral therapy (CBT) appears to have been the treatment of choice for anger over the last two decades.

A recent meta-analysis (Beck & Fernandez, 1998b) of 50 nomothetic studies of 1640 subjects receiving CBT for anger produced a weighted mean effect size of .70. This is indicative of moderate efficacy. The effect size shows that the average subject in the CBT condition was better off than 76% of control subjects. This effect was significantly different from chance, robust enough to be unaffected by unpublished null results, and relatively homogeneous across the sample of studies. The populations investigated included abusive parents or spouses, violent and resistant juvenile offenders, inmates in detention facilities, and aggressive school children. The efficacy of CBT for anger in such clinical populations raises hopes for its generalizability as a treatment for anger in pain patients.

CBAT. Given its utility in relieving residual anger, affective remediation may be included alongside cognitive and behavioral techniques for regulating anger. As expounded by Fernandez (1999, 2001), this is not merely an integrative package but an integrative program since it dictates the use of a different set of techniques at the onset, progression, and residual phases of anger. Such an integrative program of cognitive behavioural affective therapy (CBAT) is now being implemented for clinical populations known to be at risk of anger. There is good reason to believe that this CBAT program may serve a useful function in regulating anger and distress in chronic pain patients as well.

A few caveats are in order here. First of all, the objective of CBAT is not to abolish anger but to regulate it. Anger is not all dysfunctional. Besides, the inhibition of anger can be as deleterious to the individual as the overexpression of anger. As implicit in the term anger regulation, the aim is to find an *optimal* level where anger is least problematic. Also, clinicians should be aware that anger-regulation techniques might be mismatched with chronic pain patients whose anger is a byproduct of pain itself and nothing more. However, in the more common scenario of anger attributed to the actions of health professionals, significant others, or insurance companies, the same anger regulation techniques for pain-free individuals would be appropriate here.

Treatment Responsiveness and Prognosis

Fernandez and Turk (1995) have speculated that one way in which anger affects the outcome of pain treatment is through its effects on the therapeutic alliance. As emphasized in the psychotherapy literature, this alliance consists of positive regard between therapist and client and a meeting of the minds on the fundamental goals and modus operandi of therapy. Such a bond has been shown to be imperative for therapeutic success in almost any school of psychotherapy (Horvath & Symonds, 1991). This may be especially so in the context of chronic pain rehabilitation where patients are often expected to alter their very mindset about pain and to undertake behavior changes that may be counterintuitive to them. How can the therapist get the patient to exercise, reduce pain medications, and stop complaining if the patient harbors or releases anger toward the clinician? Not only will the treatment goals backfire under such circumstances, the patient's anger may be met with reciprocal anger and disinvestment on the part of the clinician. In the event of such countertransferential reactions, the already weakened working alliance is likely to collapse altogether.

Only recently has empirical research begun to verify the effect of anger on treatment outcome in pain patients. In a study by Burns et al. (1998b), 101 patients with chronic musculoskeletal pain completed a five-day-a-week multidisciplinary pain management program lasting a total of four weeks. Designed to improve both physical and psychological functioning, the program involved physical therapy, occupational therapy, cognitive-behavioral therapy at the individual and group levels, biofeedback, education, and treatment by a physician. No significant relationship was found between treatment outcome and any measure of anger for female patients. However, among the males, anger-out was negatively associated with functional capacity as measured by isoinertial lifting and treadmill walking, and anger-in was negatively correlated with general activity and depressed mood. The implication is that in multidisciplinary pain treatment, the prognosis (for males at least) is made worse by anger suppression or by anger overexpression.

This picture is rounded off by a further study (Burns et al. 1999) in which anger in pain patients affected their working alliance with health care professionals. A sample of 71 male patients who had sustained musculoskeletal injuries on the job participated in five to seven weeks of "work-hardening" designed to enhance physical, occupational, and psychosocial functioning. Just over a week into the program, patients and clinicians independently completed the Working Alliance Inventory (Tracey & Kokotovic, 1989). Results showed that neither of the measures of working alliance was related to pain duration or number of pain-related surgeries, but patients' ratings of the working alliance reached significant negative correlations with anger out (as measured by the Anger Expression Scale) and scores on the Cook-Medley Hostility scale. Interestingly, therapist perceptions of the working alliance were unrelated to anger or hostility. The two independent scores on working alliance were only marginally related. These findings suggest that even though clinicians may maintain a level of professional obligation to the angry pain patient, there is unilateral damage to the patient's part of the alliance when pain patients harbor anger at health professionals.

Conclusion

Okifuji, Turk, and Curran express some dissatisfaction with the state of research on anger and pain: "The relatively fruitless debate over the cause-effect relationship between anger and pain is reminiscent of the arguments on the associations between pain and depression (1999, p.2). Indeed the research on pain and depression has been confusing on the issue of which causes which. However, as shown in an earlier chapter, a critical synthesis of the literature does shed light on the question of causality. As for the pain-anger literature, it seems to be in a state of relative infancy and therefore sufficient research has not accumulated to enable closure on these questions. Moroever, as with the pain-depression literature, the question of causality must be placed within the broader context of multiple dynamic interactions between pain and affect. Part of the conflicting findings in the past are due to the failure to differentiate more complex interactions in which affect may act as precursor, predisposing factor, co-occurrent, exacerbator, consequence, or perpetuator of pain. Now that these models of interaction are in place and the literature reorganized accordingly, the prospect of further explicating the link between pain and affect is better than ever.

CHAPTER 6

Conclusions and Future Considerations

The word pain conjures up notions of injury or damage to the body. Occurrences of tissue damage are detected and transmitted neurologically through a process called nociception. The nociceptive signal is encoded and experienced as a physical sensation further organized into perception. Subsequent interpretation and transformation of this information proceeds during cognition. The cognitive appraisals are responsible for subjective feelings grouped under the term affect. Affect has valence, which, in the case of pain, is invariably negative or unpleasant. Affect also carries a certain intensity of arousal to support the motivation required for the organism to act in adaptive ways. This action or behavior is the cumulative and observable product of all the foregoing processes.

Typically, then, pain involves: tissue damage, nociception, sensation, perception, cognition, affect, motivation, and behavior. Of these, only sensation and affect can be regarded as defining characteristics. There are numerous exceptions to the old rule equating pain with actual tissue damage, though our immediate tendency may be to attribute our pain to injury. This explains the current definition of pain as an unpleasant sensation associated with tissue damage. The word "associated" here may be viewed in probabilistic terms to mean "with varying frequency". It may also be taken to mean that the person in pain associates it with tissue damage. This connotation with tissue damage is what distinguishes pain from other unpleasant sensations such as nausea and vertigo. It has been the objective of this book to explore the much-neglected affective component of pain. This domain extends beyond mere unpleasantness to suffering; it covers a variety of negative emotions, tonic mood states, traits, and affective disorders.   In the pain literature, three affective types have attracted the bulk of attention: depression, anxiety, and (to a lesser extent) anger.   This is mirrored across the field of mental health where anxiety, depression, and anger are of paramount interest.   These three types are referred to as the core of negative affect – and that has been the focus of the present book.

Separate chapters were devoted to each of the three core affective types as they relate to pain.   However, a common framework was used to organize the existing literature in these three areas while also opening up new areas for further research. Within this framework, six primary relationships between affect and pain were considered: affect as co-occurent, predisposing factor, precipitant, exacerbating factor, consequence, and perpetuating factor, respectively.   In other words, anxiety, depression, and anger were evaluated not merely as static correlates of pain but as dynamically interactive with pain.   These interactions were not restricted to simple cause-effect relationships but included complex modulating influences that might be exerted between each affective quality and pain.

Anxiety and Pain

In the chapter on anxiety and pain, anxiety was conceptualized in terms of the basic emotion of fear with its cognitive, behavioral and physiological features.   Pain-related fear is fueled by cognitive appraisals of danger about a variety of scenarios e.g., fear that the pain may recur, that it may be disempowering, or that it signals tissue damage, disfigurement, or even death.

Anxiety may be viewed as a problem by virtue of the intrinsic unpleasantness of fear and the obvious discomfort that comes with bodily reactions during anxiety (e.g., trembling, shaking, hyperventilating).   In the long run, anxiety-based overactivation of the sympathetic nervous system is deleterious to health.   Anxiety becomes a particularly significant problem in pain patients when it motivates chronic escape and avoidance behavior that may lead to lack of exercise, degeneration of tissue and increased sensitivity to pain. The anxiety can be so severe as to deter the individual from seeking help. In general, anxiety prognosticates poor adjustment to chronic pain and illness, and poor response to treatment. It can also turn into a burden shared by significant others who vicariously experience anxiety or else become drained of their capacity to provide constant reassurance.

When anxiety and its associated features significantly impair daily functioning, a diagnosis of anxiety disorder is appropriate. Of the dozen anxiety disorders listed, those of special relevance to pain are specific phobia, panic disorder, and generalized anxiety disorder.

Epidemiological research has revealed that the most common anxiety disorder in chronic pain is generalized anxiety disorder, with a prevalence rate of 15% in this population, followed by agoraphobia with panic attacks and simple phobia (2%). If adjustment disorder with anxious mood is thrown into the mix, the prevalence of clinical anxiety in chronic pain sufferers reaches about 60%. Chest pain and cancer pain have been of particular concern as sources of anxiety because of their association with life-threatening circumstances. Experimental pain has been minimally anxiety-provoking because of the safe and controlled conditions under which it is usually administered.

The prevalence statistic, which may be taken as an index of co-occurrence, tells us that anxiety and pain are closely related in frequency. Correlational studies go a step further by measuring the strength of association between measures of anxiety and measures of pain. As reviewed in Chapter 3, the majority of clinical research reveals a significant positive correlation between the two, though numerically, that coefficient tends to be small-to-moderate in size.

Beyond static correlations are dynamic interactions between anxiety and pain. As a predisposing factor, anxious personality traits may increase the likelihood of pain. Such dispositional variables have predicted a variety of experimentally induced pain reports and some types of clinical pain e.g., shoulder pain, dysmenorrhea, thoracic pain. Signal detection theory studies indicate that this effect is probably mediated by response bias rather than greater neural sensitivity. Trait anxiety has also been found to be a feature of hypochondriasis and somatoform pain disorder.

In contrast to the distal effect of trait anxiety on pain, a proximal effect can be exerted by state anxiety on pain. Anxious episodes last a short while during which time they act as triggers of pain. Findings on this issue vary according to the methodology used. One striking example is chest pain (in the absence of heart disease) which is triggered by panic.

The anxiety shortly before surgery predicts the level of pain that lingers after surgery. This has been observed in the context of labor pain, but not in experimental pain conditions when the source of anxiety is irrelevant to pain. Path analysis and structural equation modeling have added support to the idea that anxiety precipitates pain. However, preoperative anxiety accounts for only a small portion of the variance in postoperative pain.

Anxiety can also aggravate a pre-existing level of pain. There has been a dearth of research in this area, but clinical anecdotes leave little doubt that an individual's pain is heightened by the entry of anxiety into the picture. This is also indirectly supported by observations of diminished pain under conditions of relaxation.

Just as anxiety may intensify pain, it may also prolong the duration of pain. Pain may become stretched out in time by anxiety, especially if the anxiety is reinforced by solicitous responses from significant others. Much evidence exists for the reinforcing effect of solicitude on pain, but this is yet to be related to the underlying fear on the part of the patient.

Anxiety has been shown to accompany pain especially when the pain is perceived as a signal of disease progression or impending death. This has been witnessed in cancer patients and in cardiac pain patients. It can also occur when acute pain is shrouded in uncertainty and confusion.

The precise interface between anxiety and pain has been the subject of some postulation. One psychological viewpoint is that the negative anticipation that accompanies anxiety increases the likelihood of reporting pain. Thus, almost by self-fulfilling prophecy, anticipated pain comes to produce perceived pain.

The mechanism linking anxiety and pain may also be attentional. When anxious, there is a tendency for one to become hypervigilant and obsessional and this means a greater awareness of the slightest amount of pain. Such an explanation fits with several findings of overpredicted pain on the part of anxious individuals.

Signal detection theory experiments demonstrate that anxiety lowers an individual's criterion for pain reports. This response bias outweighs the contribution of neural sensitivity in reporting pain.

Among the biological mechanisms linking anxiety and pain, muscle tension and vascular factors have received consider-able amount of attention. The former have been implicated in musculoskeletal pain and the latter have been deemed important in migraine. Speculation has also extended to the role of hormones and endorphins in the interaction between anxiety and pain.

Clinically, numerous options have emerged to quantify and diagnose anxiety. These include unidimensional rating scales, standardized questionnaires, behavioral checklists, and psycho-physiological measures. A common choice has been a self-report questionnaire that differentiates situational from dispositional anxiety. However, there is a new generation of instruments for assessing pain-specific anxiety. Some of these are still undergoing psychometric refinement but they have the potential for more content validity when assessing issues of anxiety unique to the pain population.

Psychological interventions have been widely researched as part of a quest for safe and effective methods of regulating anxiety. Strategies such as information-giving have been shown to counter anxiety during labor and various surgical procedures. Attention-diversion has been employed in similar situations, often enhanced by hypnosis, and attaining satisfactory outcomes for children with anxiety and pain. Thought-stopping has been attempted but is of limited value when used by itself. A more elaborate cognitive technique is reappraisal. Such reinterpretation is usually guided by an astute clinician who, among many things, corrects distorted ideation about the danger of pain. The behavioral treatment of anxiety in pain patients revolves mainly around respiratory regulation, muscle relaxation, and biofeedback-assisted relaxation. Also attracting interest are touch, massage, and music. Surprisingly, systematic desensitization and exposure therapy, which have surpassed nearly all other anxiety-reducing techniques in efficacy, have been rarely attempted for pain patients with anxiety. Many techniques listed above have been integrated in an effort to maximize efficacy of anxiety control. Stress Inoculation is a prime example in this regard. Other packages have combined two or more of the following: social modeling, covert reinforcement, stimulus control, problem solving, etc.

The medications most commonly used in treating anxiety belong to a group of drugs called benzodiazepines. These have been valuable in managing the anxiety of acute pain. However, particular anxiety disorders such as phobias, panic disorder, and generalized anxiety disorder (which are known to occur in pain patients) respond differently to the various benzodiazepines. These drugs are among the safest of anxiolytics, but they are not without the risk of tolerance or other side effects. Furthermore, they tend to reduce anxiety at doses that also produce sedation. This should be carefully weighed against the need for exercise and functional restoration especially in chronic pain patients.

Depression and Pain

At the core of depression are subjective feelings of sadness. When these feelings become profound or sustained, combined with biobehavioral symptoms, and deleterious to the individual's functioning, they are regarded as clinically significant.   Different nosologies use contrasting labels for depression, but there is a consensus about two main types: major depression which is intense and episodic and dysthymia which is mild and tonic. Depressive manifestations may also occur as part of an adjustment disorder.

The idea that those in pain might also be depressed has been around for a long time, and epidemiological research has attempted to quantify this comorbidity.   Unfortunately, the prevalence statistics for depression in the pain population have been highly inconsistent, ranging anywhere from 0% to 100%. This is probably due, in large part, to sampling variations.

In this book, prevalence data on depression in pain were analyzed from two angles. First of all, the depression of pain sufferers was compared to the depression in non-pain populations. This allowed some determination of the extent to which pain is the contributing factor in depression. Secondly, greater order was achieved by separating the highly variable prevalence statistics according to homogeneous categories of pain.

Some of the important results that emerge are as follows:- in the community at large, depressive disorders are found in 2-9% of people. In the chronic pain population, the rates have been generally estimated at about 30-40%. What is interesting is that these rates in pain patients also exceed those in the primary care population but are not much different from those of medical inpatients. As explained in Chapter 4, this suggests there are many aspects of morbidity (apart from pain) that account for depression in the medically ill.

Within the pain population, the prevalence of depression shows a trend of increase from non-referred pain sufferers to patients in pain clinics. This parallels the findings of mounting depression as pain progresses from the acute to the chronic phase. There is also consistent evidence of a greater prevalence of depression in female rather than male pain patients, and an increased prevalence of depression as pain patients age. Of the various types of pain, head pain is associated with the highest rates of depression.

The subjective feelings of sadness that occur with depression are instrinsically unpleasant, and the somatic symptoms such as insomnia are clearly a source of discomfort to the individual. Anhedonia, and anergia that often occur with depression bring great functional decline in recreation, social activity, occupational responsibilities and even self-care. Depression taken to an extreme raises the further risk of self-destructiveness; in fact, it is linked to increased mortality in medical populations. It also imposes a major burden on significant others and the health care system.

The relationship between depression and pain is indexed not only by comorbidity and prevalence data but also by correlation coefficients. In the case of pain intensity, the correlation is usually moderate whereas in the case of pain duration, it tends to be smaller. Of course, there are further variations according to type of pain, but generally the pain-depression correlation coefficient is in the range of .40 to .50.

As in the case of anxiety, depression can be viewed not merely as a static correlate but as a phenomenon involved in dynamic exchange with pain. One form of such interaction is when depressive traits predispose a person to pain. This is particularly emphasized by some scholars in the psychodynamic tradition. More recent research has found less evidence for pain predisposed by depressive personality traits than by depressive mood states.

The proximal effect of a depressive episode on pain has been inferred in many studies. However, in one of the few prospective designs in this area, it was found that structural equation modeling revealed the depression-pain link to be far weaker than the pain-depression link.

The possible aggravating effect of depression on pre-existing pain has also been investigated. Most of the studies in this area have employed experimental pain induction. In this context, it has been shown that depressed individuals tend to have higher pain thresholds than non-depressed counterparts. This is in stark contrast to the intensifying effect of anxiety on pain. The decreased pain sensitivity in depressives has been attributed to lowered sensory discrimination plus an increased bias against reporting pain.

A possible role of depression in perpetuating pain has been considered by psychoanalysts. They invoke a compensatory principle to explain how pain is sustained over time by feelings of helplessness. Learning theory explains this by reinforcement principles whereby pain behaviors may persist as a function of the solicitous behaviors elicited by helplessness and depression.

Perhaps the strongest link between pain and depression is evident when pain is viewed as the causal antecedent. As mentioned earlier, structural equation modeling in the context of a prospective study has revealed that the causal role of pain in depression outweighs the reverse by which depression causes pain. Additional research has demonstrated that the previous day's pain predicts the present day's depression.

Finally, much attention has been devoted to the concept of pain as masked depression. One postulation here is that some depressives are alexithymic and therefore likely to express themselves through bodily reactions like pain. Another idea is that pain serves as a cover-up for depression in those who are reluctant to be viewed as psychiatrically disturbed. Despite much conjecture to it, the pain-as-masked depression hypothesis has received little empirical support.

In the search for a mechanism to explain the pain-depression relationship, scholars have adopted a variety of biological and psychosocial viewpoints. These were reviewed in Chapter 4 under the categories of: genetic family studies, symptom overlap, common biological markers, common personality traits, cognitive styles, cognitive distortions, life interference, helplessness, and reinforcement contingencies. Evidence on some of these is unconvincing, and in other cases it is strong. Still, it may be wise to accommodate more than one viewpoint into the etiology of pain and depression. One attempt to do so is the diathesis-stress theory. This theory is compelling in some ways, but (as discussed) it is not without shortcomings when explaining some of the epidemiological intricacies in pain and depression.

The clinical assessment of depression has been dominated by self-report methods, though the search for biological markers continues.   Most commonly used are four depression scales, though more concise versions of these have been used in pain patients. A host of subscales from comprehensive instruments are also available for assessing depression in pain patients. Whatever the instrument used, it is of utmost importance to keep in mind that pain patients' scores on these scales may be inflated by physical symptoms (e.g., sleep disturbance, motor slowing, and appetite change) that are the product of pain rather than depression. Some correction methods were suggested to handle this confounding of somatic-behavioral and cognitive-affective symptoms of depression in pain sufferers. Other measurement issues discussed were cultural appropriateness, diagnostic documentation practices, and the peculiarities of retrospective data.

The form of psychological treatment for depression has ranged from cognitive and psychodynamic techniques for reappraising depressive ideation to behavior modification and kinesthetic methods including exercise. There has been a modicum of interest in experiential and emotive therapies centered around the expression of inhibited affect. Of particular note is that in the pain population, evidence has emerged for patterns of cognitive distortions which diminish or weaken with reappraisal and coping techniques.

If diagnosed with depression, pain patients might receive a course of antidepressant medications. Four major classes of such medications were described, of which the most preferred seem to be the tricyclics. One question of interest to many researchers is whether these medications have an analgesic effect or a mood-elevating effect.   When studies addressing this issue were organized along two dimensions (diagnosis and drug effect) it was found that the bulk of evidence favored an antidepressant rather than an analgesic effect of these drugs. This outcome was further qualified by other factors such as expectancy variables, toxicity, and side effects.

Anger and Pain

Though much neglected in research on pain, anger is one of the modal emotions and a key element in the core of negative affect. By mobilizing the organism to the fight response, it is one of a repertoire of adaptive responses to aversive stimuli such as pain. Chapter 5 began with the conceptualization of anger as an emotion comprising appraisals of wrongdoing and motivations to aggression. Anger was distinguished from hostility, frustration and other related terms. Work is only just beginning on the different types of affective disorders that may have anger as their primary emotion.

Social psychological surveys indicate that about two-thirds of the community report anger about once or twice a week. A few researchers have also begun to highlight anger in the chronically ill. In a study sponsored by the World Health Organization, anger outstripped anxiety and sadness to become the most common concern affecting almost 80% of those with weekly back pain, headache, or abdominal pain. Recent research has revealed that much of this anger is indeed pain-related -- a majority of pain patients being angry with their health care providers while many are also angry with their significant others and themselves. No appreciable gender differences have been found for anger in pain sufferers.

The adverse effects of anger are not merely confined to the obvious aggression and destruction commonly attributed to this emotion. Anger also mars interpersonal relations, and when inhibited it can turn into depression. A wave of research has accumulated in support of the idea that angry people are prone to cardiovascular disease and that they are likely to adopt unhealthy habits. Of specific relevance to the pain population is the observation that anger also interferes with the therapeutic alliance so vital to the management of pain.

As with anxiety and depression, anger is related to pain in multiple ways. First of all, it can be represented as a simple correlate. Anger levels have been found to be positively associated with pain report, pain behaviors, and pain-related disability.

Secondly, like other affective traits, hostility might be viewed as a predisposing factor in pain. However, the few studies that have made claims along these lines are based on correlational analyses.

There is some evidence for the role of anger as a precipitant of pain. The experimental induction of anger has been found to increase pain of migraine as well as tension headache.

The remaining three models of interaction stipulate that anger might also function as an aggravating factor, perpetuating factor, or consequence of pain. However, the literature on anger and pain is still in its infancy and there is little evidence that could be brought to bear on these possibilities. These are not grounds for discarding these models of anger and pain. Understandably, in time to come, more empirical data will accumulate to permit tests of these hypotheses just as data has allowed tests of the inter-actions between pain and other affective qualities.

The underlying mechanism linking pain and anger has been explained primarily with reference to cognitive appraisal theory of emotions. Anger is not simply a hardwired reaction to aversive stimuli or a function of autonomic arousal. In the present context, it is governed by active interpretation of pain and its associated circumstances. Thus, the person in chronic pain is inclined to get angry with medical health care providers for treatment failures, with mental health professionals for any suggestion of psycho-pathology, with significant others for lack of emotional or material support, and with many others for reasons detailed in Chapter 5. The actions of these agents, when construed as wrongful or neglectful, are what subserve anger. Of course, this does not discount the possibility that sympathetic nervous system arousal increases the intensity of anger and pain.

The tools of choice in the clinical assessment of anger and hostility are self-report tests, although these are increasingly supplemented with behavioral observations and self-monitoring techniques. Described in Chapter 5 were several self-report tests that use hypothetical scenarios, or self-descriptive statements that patients respond to. At least one test stood out by virtue of its distinction between state versus trait anger, and anger-in versus anger-out. New efforts to develop tools for assessing the targets and reasons for anger in pain patients were also described.

Because anger is less socially acceptable than depression and anxiety, it is often supressed so as to elude even clinicians. Besides, the item content of tests of anger is often transparent so that test-takers are able to respond in ways that conceal this emotion. Fortunately, there are tests of social presentation bias that may be included in any battery of anger measures. These allow the clinician to make more valid inferences about the anger of pain patients.

The treatment of anger has been almost exclusively cognitive-behavioral in orientation. Reappraisal through rational disputation and coping statements is at the heart of this approach. In the case of anger-related arousal, the many relaxation techniques indicated for anxiety are also applicable here. Behavior modification through contracts, stimulus control, and rehearsal are also beneficial as anger prevention techniques. Finally, new efforts are underway to revive the use of cathartic techniques under the general rubric of expressive or experiential therapy. These techniques may be particularly suited to what is called residual anger.

Future Considerations

There is a need to study affect not only as a static correlate of pain but as a phenomenon that interacts dynamically with pain. These dynamics go beyond simple cause-effect relations; they include predisposing, precipitating, aggravating, consequential, and perpetuating roles of affect in pain. Future investigations might help fill the current vacuum of evidence for some of these functions in particular areas of pain research. Research is also needed to pit the above interactions against one another -- much like competing hypotheses about the relationship between affect and pain.

There is a need for greater differentiation among types of pain as they relate to types of affect. The vagaries of epidemiological findings on pain and depression alert us to the need to organize such data according to different pain disorders. Affect itself can be further differentiated into subtypes. Even though anger, fear, and sadness constitute the core of negative affect, the emotional, temperamental, and dispositional variants of these may relate differently to pain. The affective disorders of anxiety, depressive and anger disorders can also be classified into diagnostic subtypes which need not be similar in the way they interact with pain.

This book has shown that certain demographic factors moderate or qualify the links between affect and pain. However, more research is needed to explore how males and females differ, particularly in the experience versus expression of affect. It is apparent that there are age-related differences in the relative prominence of anxiety, depression, and anger in pain sufferers, but what is sorely missing here is a life span developmental perspective. Similarly, ethnic subgroups have been studied, but usually in isolation from one another. What would be more informative would be cross-cultural comparisons. This is important because the very diagnoses of anxiety, depression and anger disorders are made with reference to prevailing sociocultural norms.

As for the underlying mechanisms by which affect and pain are linked, biological and psychosocial etiologies have been advanced. However, these appear to have been developed without much appreciation for how these mechanisms might themselves be connected at some level. A unifying theory may be a distant prospect but there is enough evidence to begin building the foundations of a biopsychosocial theory of affect in pain.

The assessment of affect in pain sufferers has been somewhat narrow, with most clinicians relying on a few self-report tests as a matter of convenience or convention. New psychometric tests are constantly appearing, as are specific tests for assessment of affect in the pain population. The incremental utility of these instruments needs to be evaluated. Psychometrically sound instruments, alike other methods of affect measurement, are not definitive. Therefore, they should be corroborated with data from alternative assessment tools. Of special value in the assessment of affect is the inclusion of naturalistic behavioral observations to circumvent the reactivity of clinical testing, validity tests to help correct for social desirability bias, and biochemical indices of the arousal and intensity of affect.

The treatment of negative affect in pain patients has fallen within two broad categories: cognitive behavioral therapy and psychotropic medication. These two approaches have occasionally been combined, but for the most part, the literature in this area remains divided. An additional limitation is the insufficient tailoring of techniques to problems. Against the backdrop of models relating affect and pain, it is now timely to match treatment techniques to the particular pain-affect dynamic. For example, affective traits might respond best to characterological therapies, affective episodes that precipitate pain may be handled by immediate cognitive intervention, and residual affective consequences of chronic pain might diminish with expressive therapies. For some problems such as anger, it may be necessary to select different techniques suited to the prevention, intervention, and remediation of affect, respectively. This kind of technical selectivism is more promising than technical eclecticism when there is some clarity about diagnosis or etiology. Where the mechanism or etiology of affect is obfuscated, an integrative approach to treatment may maximize the likelihood of a favorable outcome; one option in this regard is CBAT or cognitive behavioural affective therapy. Ultimately, selectivism and integrationism also depend on a certain amount of innovation in treatment. Much progress has been witnessed in the treatment of anxiety, depression, and anger in pain patients, but new developments would bring an even greater degree of freedom and success to this endeavor.

References

Abramson, L. Y., Seligman, M. E., & Teasdale, J. D. (1978). Learned helplessness in humans: Critique and reformulation. *Journal of Abnormal Psychology, 87,* 49-74.

Abraham, K. (1911). Notes on the psychoanalytic investigation and treatment of manic-depressive insanity and allied conditions. In: *Selected papers on psychoanalysis.* London: Hogarth press.

Abraham, K. (1924). A short study of the development of the libido viewed in the light of mental disorders. In: *Selected Papers of psychoanalysis.* London: Hogarth Press.

Achterberg, J., Kenner, C., & Casey, D. (1989). Behavioral strategies for the reduction of pain and anxiety associated with orthopedic trauma. *Biofeedback & Self Regulation, 14,* 101-114.

Achterberg-Lawlis, J. (1982). The psychological dimensions of arthritis. *Journal of Consulting and Clinical Psychology, 50,* 984-992.

Ackerman, M. D., & Stevens, M. J. (1989). Acute and chronic pain: Pain dimensions and psychological status. *Journal of Clinical Psychology. 45,* 223-228.

Affleck, G., Tennen, H., Urrows, S., & Higgins, P. (1991). Individual differences in the day-to-day experience of chronic pain: A prospective daily study of rheumatoid arthritis patients. *Health Psychology, 10,* 419-426.

Affleck, G., Urrows, S., Tennen, H., Higgins, P., et al. (1996). Sequential daily relations of sleep, pain intensity, and attention to pain among women with fibromyalgia. *Pain, 68,* 363-368.

Ahles, T.A., Ruckdeschel, J.C., & Blanchard, E.B. Cancer-related pain: II. (1984). Assessment with Visual Analogue Scales. *Journal of Psychosomatic Research. 28,* 121-124.

Akiskal, H. S. (1981). Subaffective disorders: Dysthymic, cyclothymic, and bipolar II disorders in the "borderline" realm. *Psychiatric Clinics of North America, 4*, 25-46.

Akiskal, H. S. (1996). Dysthymia as a temperamental variant of affective disorder. *European Psychiatry, 11*, 117s-122s.

Al Absi, M. & Rokke, P. D. Can anxiety help us tolerate pain? (1991). *Pain. 46*, 43-51.

Allodi, F., & Goldstein, R. (1995). Posttraumatic somatoform disorders among immigrant workers. *Journal of Nervous and Mental Disease, 183*, 604-607.

Almay, B. G., et al. (1978). Endorphins in chronic pain: I. Differences in CSF endorphin levels between organic and psychogenic pain syndromes. *Pain, 5*, 153-162.

American Psychiatric Association (1980*). Diagnostic and Statistical Manual of Mental Disorders Third Edition (DSM-III).* Washington, D.C.: American Psychiatric Association.

American Psychiatric Association (2000). *Diagnostic and statistical manual of mental disorders Fourth Edition Text Revision (DSM-IV-TR).* Washington, D.C.: American Psychiatric Association.

Anderson, K. O., Keefe, F. J., Bradley, L. A., McDaniel, L. K. et al (1988). Prediction of pain behavior and functional status of rheumatoid arthritis patients using medical status and psychological variables. *Pain, 33*, 25-32.

Andreasen, N. C. (1987). The measurement of genetic aspects of depression. In A.J. Marsella, R.M.A. Hirschfeld & M.M. Katz (Eds.). *The measurement of depression* (pp. 87- 108). New York: Guilford.

Aneshensel, C. S., Frerichs, R. R., & Huba, G. J. (1984). Depression and physical illness: A multiwave, nonrecursive causal model. *Journal of Health & Social Behavior, 25*, 350-371.

Arana, G. W., Teicher, M. H., & Baldessarini, R. J. "The utility of the dexamethasone suppression test": In reply. *Archives of General Psychiatry, 44,* 95-96.

Arieti S. (1962). The psychotherapeutic approach to depression. *American Journal of Psychotherapy, 16,* 397 - 406.

Arieti, S., & Bemporad, J. (1978). *Severe and mild depression: The psychotherapeutic approach.* New York: Basic Books.

Arnstein, P., Caudill, M., Mandle, C. L., Norris, A., & Beasley, R. (1999). Self efficacy as a mediator of the relationship between pain intensity, disability and depression in chronic pain patients. *Pain, 80,* 483-491.

Arntz, A., & de Jong, P. F. (1993). Anxiety, attention and pain. *Journal of Psychosomatic Research. 37,* 423-431.

Arntz, A., Dreessen, L., & De Jong, P. (1994). The influence of anxiety on pain: Attentional and attributional mediators. *Pain, 56,* 307-314.

Arntz, A., Van Eck, M., & Heijmans, M. (1990). Predictions of dental pain: The fear of any expected evil is worse than the evil itself. *Behaviour Research & Therapy, 28,* 29-41.

Arntz, A., Dreessen, L., & Merckelbach, H. (1991). Attention, not anxiety, influences pain. *Behaviour Research & Therapy, 29,* 41-50.

Aronoff, G. M., & Evans, W. O. (1982). Doxepin as an adjunct in the treatment of chronic pain. *Journal of Clinical Psychiatry, 43,* 42 – 47.

Aronoff, G. M., Wagner, J. M. & Spangler, A. S., (1986). Chemical interventions of pain. *Journal of Consulting and Clinical Psychology, 54,* 769 -775.

Asmundson, G. J. G., & Norton, G. (1995). Anxiety sensitivity in patients with physically unexplained chronic back pain: A preliminary report. *Behaviour Research & Therapy, 33,* 771-777.

Asmundson, G. J. G., & Taylor, S. (1996). Role of anxiety sensitivity in pain-related fear and avoidance. *Journal of Behavioral Medicine. 19,* 577-586.

Asmundson, G. J. G., Frombach, I. K., & Hadjistavropoulos, H. D. (1998). Anxiety sensitivity: Assessing factor structure and relationship to multidimensional aspects of pain in injured workers. *Journal of Occupational Rehabilitation, 8,* 223-234.

Asmundson, G. J. G., Norton, P. J., & Norton, G. R. (1999). Beyond pain: The role of fear and avoidance in chronicity. *Clinical Psychology Review. 19,* 97-119.

Atkinson, J. H., Slater, M. A., Patterson, T. L., & Grant, I. (1991). Prevalence, onset, and risk of psychiatric disorders in men with chronic low back pain: A controlled study. *Pain, 45,* 111-121.

Averill, J. R. (1982). *Anger and aggression: An essay on emotion.* New York: Springer-Verlag.

Averill, P. M., Novy, D. M., Nelson, D. V., & Berry, L. A. (1996). Correlates of depression in chronic pain patients: A comprehensive examination. *Pain, 65,* 93 - 100.

Azrin, N. H., & Besalel, V. A. (1982). An operant reinforcement method of treating depression. *Journal of Behavior therapy and Experimental Psychiatry, 12,* 145-151.

Bancroft, J., & Rennie, D. (1995). Perimenstrual depression: Its relationship to pain, bleeding and pervious history of depression. *Psychosomatic Medicine, 57,* 445-452.

Bancroft, J., Williamson, L., & Warner, P. (1993). Perimenstrual complaints in women complaining of PMS, menorrhagia and dysmenorrhoea: Towards a dismantling of the premenstrual syndrome. *Psychosomatic Medicine, 55,* 133-145.

Bandura, A. (1977). *Social learning theory.* Englewood Cliffs, NJ: Prentice-Hall.

Banks, S. M., & Kerns, R. D. (1996). Explaining high rates of depression in chronic pain: A diathesis-stress framework. *Psychological Bulletin, 119,* 95-110.

Barefoot, J. C. (1992). Developments in the measurement of hostility. In H.S. Friedman (Ed.), *Hostility, coping and health* (pp.13-31). Washington, D.C.: American Psychological Association.

Barefoot, J. C., Dahlstrom, W. G., & Williams, R.B.Jr. (1983). Hostility, CHD incidence, and total mortality. A 25-year follow-up study of 255 physicians. *Psychosomatic Medicine, 45,* 59-63.

Barlow, D. H., & Brown, T. A. (1996). Psychological treatments for panic disorder and panic disorder with agoraphobia. In M.R. Mavissakalian & Prien (Eds.), *Long-term treatments of anxiety disorders* (pp.221-240). Washington, DC: American Psychiatric Press, Inc.

Barlow, D. H., Craske, M. G., Cerny, J. A., & Klosko, J.S. (1989). Behavioral treatment of panic disorder. *Behavior Therapy, 20,* 261-282.

Baron, R. A. (1977). *Human aggression.* New York: Plenum.

Basbaum, A., & Fields, H. L. (1978). Endogenous pain control mechanisms: Review and hypothesis. *Annals of Neurology, 4,* 451 – 462.

Basbaum, A. I., & Fields, H. L. (1980). The reticular formation revisited. In J.A. Hopsonand & M. A. B. Brazier (Eds.), *Pain control: A new role for the medullary reticular formation.* New York: Raven Press.

Basler, H. D., & Rehfisch, H. P. (1990). Follow-up results of a cognitive-behavioural treatment for chronic pain in a primary care setting. *Psychology & Health, 4,* 293-304.

Bateson, A. N. (2002). Basic pharmacologic mechanisms involved in benzodiazepine tolerance and withdrawal. *Current Pharmaceutical Design, 8,* 5-21.

Baumstark, K. E., Buckelew, S. P., Sher, K. J., Beck, N., Buescher, K. L., Hewett, J., & Crews, T. M. (1993). Pain behavior predictors among fibromyalgia patients. *Pain, 55,* 339-346.

Bayer, T. L., Chiang, E., Coverdale, J. H., Bangs, M. et al. (1993). Anxiety in experimentally induced somatoform symptoms. Psychosomatics. *34,* 416-423.

Beck, A. T. (1976). *Cognitive therapy and the emotional disorders.* New York: International Universities.

Beck, A. T. (1967). *Depression: Clinical, experimental, and theo-retical aspects*. New York: Harper & Row.

Beck, A. T. (1978). *Depression inventory*. Minneapolis, MN: University of Minnesota Press.

Beck, A. T. (1991). Cognitive therapy: A 30-year retrospective. *American Psychologist, 46*, 368-375.

Beck, A. T., Emery, G., & Greenberg, R. L. (1985). *Anxiety disorders and phobias: A cognitive perspective*. New York: Basic Books.

Beck, A. T., Steer, R. A., & Garbin, M. G. (1988). Psychometric properties of the Beck Depression Inventory: Twenty five years of evaluation. *Clinical Psychology Review, 8*, 77-100.

Beck, A. T., Ward, C. H., Mendelson, M., Mock, J., & Erbaugh, J. (1961). An inventory for measuring depression. *Archives of General Psychiatry, 4*, 561-571.

Beck, R., & Fernandez, E. (1998a). Cognitive-behavioral self-regulation of the frequency, duration, and intensity of anger. *Journal of Psychopathology and Behavioral Assessment, 20*, 217-229.

Beck, R., & Fernandez, E. (1998b). Cognitive-behavioral therapy in the treatment of anger: A meta-analysis. *Cognitive Therapy and Research, 22*, 63-74.

Becker, N., Thomsen, A. B., Olsen, A. K., Sjogren, P., Bech, P., & Eriksen, J. (1997). Pain epidemiology and health related quality of life in chronic non-malignant pain patients referred to a Danish multidisciplinary pain center. *Pain, 73*, 393-400.

Beck-Friis, J. (1983). Melatonin in depressive disorder. A methodological and clinical study of the pineal-hypothalamic-pituitary-adrenal cortex system. Doctoral Dissertation. Stockholm: Karolinska Institute.

Beecher, H. K. (1959). Generalization from pain of various types and diverse origins. *Science, 130*, 267-268.

Beecher, H. K. (1957). The measurement of Pain: Prototype for the quantitative study of subjective responses. *Pharmacological Reviews*, *9*, 59-209.

Beitman, B. D., DeRosear, L., Basha, I. M., Flaker, G. et al (1987). Panic disorder in cardiology patients with atypical or non-anginal chest pain: A pilot study. *Journal of Anxiety Disorders, 1*, 277-282.

Belanger, E., Melzack, R., & Lauzon, P. (1989). Pain of first-trimester abortion: A study of psychosocial and medical predictors. *Pain, 36*, 339 - 350.

Ben-Tovim, D. I., & Schwartz, M. S. (1981). Hypoalgesia in depressive illness. *British Journal of Psychiatry, 138*, 37-39.

Ben-Zur, H., & Breznitz, S. (1991). What makes people angry: Dimensions of anger provoking events. *Journal of Research in Personality, 25*, 1-22.

Berkowitz, L. (1990). On the formation and regulation of anger and aggression: A cognitive-neoassociationistic analysis. *American Psychologist, 45*, 494-503.

Berkowitz, L., & Heimer, K. (1989). On the construction of the anger experience: Aversive events and negative priming in the formation of feelings. *Advances in Experimental Social Psychology, 22*, 1-37.

Beutler, L., Engle, D., Oro'-Beutler, M., Daldrup, R., & Meredith, K. (1986). Inability to express intense affect: A common link between depression and pain? *Journal of Counseling and Clinical Psychology, 54*, 752-759.

Beutler, L. E., Daldrup, R. J. Engle, D., Oro-Beutler, M. E., Meredith, K., & Boyer, J. T. (1987). Effects of therapeutically induced affect arousal on depressive symptoms, pain, and beta-endorphins among rheumatoid arthritis patients. *Pain, 29*, 325 - 334.

Bezzi, G., Pinelli, P., & Tosca, P. (1981). Motor reactivity, pain threshold and effects of sleep deprivation in unipolar depressives. *Psychiatrica Clinica, 14*, 150-160.

Biaggio, M. K. (1980). Assessment of anger arousal. *Journal of Personality Assessment, 44*, 289-298.

Biaggio, M. K. , & Maiuro , R. D . (1985). Recent advances in anger assessment. In C. D. Spielberger & J. N. Butcher (Eds.), *Advances in personality assessment*. Hillsdale, N.J.: Lawrence Erlbaum.

Biederman, J. J., & Schefft, B. K. (1994). Behavioral, physiological, and self-evaluative effects of anxiety on the self-control of pain. *Behavior Modification, 18*, 89-105.

Blackwell, B. (1987). Side effects of antidepressant drugs. *Psychiatry Update, 6*, 724-725.

Blalock, S. J., De Vellis, R. F., Brown, G. K., & Wallston, K. A. (1989). Validity of the Center for Epidemiological Studies Depression Scale in arthritis populations. *Arthritis and Rheumatism, 32*, 991-997.

Blanchard, E. B., Andrasik, F., Neff, D. F., Arena, J. G., Ahles, T. A., Jurish, S. E., Pallmeyer, T. P. , Saunders, N. L. , Teders, S. J. , Barron, K. D. , & Rodichok, L. D. (1982). Biofeedback and relaxation training with three kinds of headache: Treatment effects and their prediction. *Journal of Consulting and Clinical Psychology, 50*, 562 - 575.

Blanco, C., Antia, S. X., & Liebowitz, M. R. (2002). Pharmacotherapy of social anxiety disorder. *Biological Psychiatry, 51*, 109-120.

Block, A. R. , Kremer, E. F. , & Gaylor, M. (1980). Behavioral treatment of chronic pain: The spouse as a discriminative cue for pain behavior. *Pain, 9*, 243-252.

Bloschl, L. (1975). Loss of reinforcement and depressive reaction: A model based on learning theory. *Archiv fuer Psychologie, 127*, 51-69.

Blumer D. & Heilbron M. (1981). Chronic pain as a variant of depressive disease: The pain-prone disorder. *Journal of Nervous and Mental Disease, 170*, 381 - 406.

Blumer D. & Heilbronn M., (1984a). Antidepressant treatment for chronic pain. *Psychiatric Annals, 14*, 796 - 800.

Blumer D. & Heilbronn M., (1984b). "Chronic pain as a variant of depressive disease": A rejoinder. *Journal of Nervous and Mental Disease, 172,* 405-407.

Blumer, D., Heilbronn, M., & Pedraza, E., et al (1980). Systematic treatment of chronic pain with antidepressants. *Henry Ford Hospital Medical Journal, 28,* 15 – 21.

Blumer, D. , Zorick, F. , Heilbronn, M. , & Roth, T. (1982). Biological markers for depression in chronic pain. *Journal of Nervous & Mental Disorder, 170,* 425-428.

Boeke, S., Duivenvoorden, H.J., Verhage, F., & Zwaveling, A. (1991). Prediction of postoperative pain and duration of hospitalization using two anxiety measures. *Pain, 45,* 293-297.

Botney, M., & Fields, H. L. (1982). Amitriptyline potentiates morphine analgesics by a direct action on the central nervous system. *Annual Neurology, 13,* 160-164.

Boureau, F., Gay, C., & Combes, A. (1990). Douleur chronique, depression et serotonine. /Chronic pain, depression and serotonin. *Psychiatrie & Psychobiologie, 5,* 169-178.

Bowen, R. C., D'Arcy, C., & Orchard, R. C. (1991). The prevalence of anxiety disorders among patients with mitral valve prolapse syndrome and chest pain. *Psychosomatics, 32,* 400-406.

Bowlby, J. (1969). *Attachment.* New York: Basic Books.

Boyle, G. J. (1985). Self-report measures of depression: Some psychometric considerations. *British Journal of Clinical Psychology, 24,* 45-59.

Boyle, G. J. , & Ciccone, V. M. (1994). Relaxation alone and in combination with rational emotive therapy: Effects on mood and pain. *The Pain Clinic, 7,* 253-265.

Bradley, J. J. (1963). Severe localized pain associated with the depressive syndrome. *British Journal of Psychiatry, 109,* 741-745.

Braha, R., & Catchlove, R. (1986). Pain and anger: Inadequate expression in chronic pain patients. *The Pain Clinic, 1,* 125-129.

Bridges, K. W. , & Goldberg, D. P. (1984). Psychiatric illness in in-patients with neurological disorders: Patients' views on discussion of emotional problems with neurologists. *British Medical Journal, 289,* 656-658.

Bridges, K. W., & Goldberg, D. P. (1985). Somatic presentation of DSM III psychiatric disorders in primary care. *Journal of Psychosomatic Research, 29,* 563-569.

Bronzo, A. Jr. , & Powers, G. (1967). Relationship of anxiety with pain threshold. *Journal of Psychology, 66,* 181-183.

Brown, G. K. (1990). A causal analysis of chronic pain and depression. *Journal of Abnormal Psychology, 99,* 127-137.

Brown, R. A., Fader, K., & Barber, T. X. (1973). Responsiveness to pain: Stimulus-specificity versus generality. *Psychological Record, 23,* 1-7.

Brown, R. T., & Jamil, K. (1993). Costochondritis in adolescents: A follow-up study. *Clinical Pediatrics, 32,* 499-500.

Bru, E., Mykletun, R. J., & Svebak, S. (1993). Neuroticism, extroversion, anxiety and Type A behaviour as mediators of neck shoulder and lower back pain in female hospital staff. *Personality & Individual Differences, 15,* 485-492.

Bruce, M. L. , & Leaf, P. J. (1989). Psychiatric disorders and 15-month mortality in a community sample of older adults. *American Journal of Public Health, 79,*727-730.

Bruegel, M. A. (1971). Relationship of preoperative anxiety to perception of postoperative pain. *Nursing Research, 20,* 26-31.

Buchwald, A. M. (1977). Depressive mood and estimates of reinforcement frequency. *Journal of Abnormal Psychology, 86,* 443-446.

Buck, R. (1985). Prime theory: An integrated view of emotion and motivation. *Psychological Review, 92,* 389-413.

Budzynski, T. H. , & Stoyva, J. M. (1969). An instrument for producing deep muscle relaxation by means of analog information feedback. *Journal of Applied Behavior Analysis, 2,* 231-237.

Buescher K. L., Johnston, J. A., Parker J. C., Smarr K. L., Buckelew S. P., Anderson S.K., & Walker S. E. (1991). *Journal of Rheumatology, 18,* 968-972.

Burns, J. W. (1997). Anger management style and hostility: Predicting symptom-specific physiological reactivity among chronic low back patients. *Journal of Behavioral Medicine, 20,* 505-522.

Burns, J. W., Higdon, L. J., Mullen, J. T. , Lansky, D., & Wei, J. M. (1999). Relationships among patient hostility, anger expression, depression, and the working alliance in a work hardening program. *Annals of Behavioral Medicine, 21,* 77-82.

Burns, J. W., Johnson, B. J., Devine, J., Mahoney, N., & Pawl, R. (1998a). Anger management style and the prediction of treatment outcome among male and female chronic pain patients. *Behaviour Research and Therapy, 36,* 1051-1062.

Burns, J. W., Johnson, B. J., Mahoney, N., Devine, J., & Pawl, R. (1998b). Cognitive and physical capacity process variables predict long-term outcome after treatment of chronic pain. *Journal of Consulting and Clinical Psychology, 66,* 434-439.

Burns, J. W. , Johnson, B. J. , Mahoney, N. , Devine, J. , & Pawl, R. (1996). Anger management style, hostility and spouse responses: Gender differences in predictors of adjustment among chronic pain patients. *Pain, 64,* 445-453.

Burns, J. W. , Wiegner, S. , Derleth, M. , Kiselica, K. , & Pawl, R. (1997). Linking symptom-specific physiological reactivity to pain severity in chronic low back pain patients: A test of mediation and moderation models. *Health Psychology, 16,* 319-326.

Bush, C., Ditto, B., & Feuerstein, M. (1985). A controlled evaluation of paraspinal EMG biofeedback in the treatment of chronic low back pain. *Health Psychology, 4,* 307-321.

Buss, A. H. (1961). *The psychology of aggression.* New York: Wiley.

Buss, A. H. , & Durkee, A. (1957). An inventory for assessing different kinds of hostility. *Journal of Consulting Psychology, 21*, 343-349.

Butcher, J. N. , Graham, J. R. , Williams, C. L. , & Ben-Porath, Y. S. (1990). *Development and use of the MMPI-2 Content Scales*. Minneapolis, MN: University of Minnesota Press.

Cacioppo, J. T. , Bernston, G. G. , Klein, D. J. & Poehlmann, K. M. (1997). The psychophysiology of emotion across the lifespan. *Annual Review of Gerontology and Geriatrics, 17*, 27-74.

Caine, T. M. , Foulds, G. A. , & Hope, K. (1967). *Manual of the hostility and direction of hostility questionnaire*. London: University of London.

Calfas, K. , Ingram, R. E. , & Kaplan, R. M. (1997). Information processing and affective distress in osteoarthritis patients. *Journal of Consulting and Clinical Psychology, 65*, 576 - 581.

Callahan L. F. , Brooks, R. H. , & Pincus, T. (1988). Further analysis of learned helplessness in rheumatoid arthritis using a "Rheumatology Attitudes Index". *Journal of Rheumatology, 15*, 418-426.

Carlson, C. R., & Curran, S. L. (1994). Stretch-based relaxation training. *Patient Education & Counseling, 23*, 5-12.

Carosso, R. L., Yehuda, S. , & Streifler, M. (1979). Clomipramine and amitriptyline in the treatment of severe pain. *International Journal of Neuroscience, 9*, 191–194.

Carter, C. S., Maddock, R. J. (1992). Chest pain in generalized anxiety disorder. *International Journal of Psychiatry in Medicine, 22*, 291-298

Carter, C. S., Servan-Schreiber, D., & Perlstein, W. M. (1997). Anxiety disorders and the syndrome of chest pain with normal coronary arteries: Prevalence and pathophysiology. *Journal of Clinical Psychiatry, 58*, 70-75.

Cartwright, A., Hockey, L., & Anderson, J. L. (1973). *Life before death*. London: Boston, Routledge and Kegan Paul.

Casten, R. J., Parmelee, P. A., Kleban, M. H., Lawton, M. P., et al (1995). The relationships among anxiety, depression, and pain in a geriatric institutionalized sample. *Pain, 61,* 271-276.

Cattell, R. B. (1965). *The scientific analysis of personality.* London, UK: Penguin.

Cavanaugh, S. V. A. (1983). The prevalence of emotional and cognitive dysfunction in a general medical population: Using the MMSE, GHQ, and BDI. *General Hospital Psychiatry, 5,* 15-24.

Channer, K. S., & Rees, J. R. (1987). Affect and angina. *Stress Medicine, 3,* 141-146.

Chapman, C. R., & Bulter, S. H. (1976). Effects of doxepin on perception of laboratory-induced pain in man. *Pain, 5,* 253 – 262.

Chapman, C. R., & Cox, G. B. (1977). Anxiety, pain, and depression surrounding elective surgery: A multivariate comparison of abdominal surgery patients with kidney donors and recipients. *Journal of Psychosomatic Research, 21,* 7-15.

Chapman, C. R., & Feather, B. W. (1973). Effects of diazepam on human pain tolerance and pain sensitivity. *Psychosomatic Medicine, 35,* 330-340.

Chapman, C. R., Dingman, H. F., & Ginzberg, S. P. (1965). Failure of systematic analgesic agents to alter the absolute sensory threshold for the simple detection of pain. *Brain, 88,* 1011-1022.

Charatan, F. B. (1975). Depression in old age. *New York State Journal of Medicine, 75,* 2505-2509.

Chaturvedi, S. K. (1987). A comparison of depressed and anxious chronic pain patients. *General Hospital Psychiatry, 9,* 383-386.

Chaturvedi, S. K. (1989). Psychalgic depressive disorder: A descriptive and comparative study. *Acta Psychiatrica Scandinavica, 79,* 98-102.

Chaturvedi, S. K., & Michael, A. (1986). Chronic pain in a psychiatric clinic. *Journal of Psychosomatic Research, 30*, 347-354.

Cheren, S. (Ed.), (1989). *Psychosomatic medicine: theory, physiology, and practice.* Madison, CT: International Universities Press.

Cipher, D. J., & Fernandez, E. (1997). Expectancy variables predicting tolerance and avoidance of pain in chronic pain patients. *Behaviour Research & Therapy, 35*, 437-444.

Cipher, D. J., Fernandez, E., & Clifford, P. A. (2001). Cost-effectiveness and health care utilization in a multidisciplinary pain center: Comparison of three treatment groups. *Journal of Clinical Psychology in Medical Settings, 8*, 237-244.

Cipher, D. J., Fernandez, E., & Clifford, P. A. (2002). Coping style influences compliance with multidisciplinary pain management. *Journal of Health Psychology, 7,* 665-673.

Clark, W. C., Yang, J. C., & Janal, M. N. (1986). Altered pain and visual sensitivity in humans: The effects of acute and chronic stress. *Annals of the New York Academy of Sciences, 467*, 116-129.

Clarke, I. M. C. (1981). Amitriptyline and perphenazine (Triptafen D.A.) in chronic pain. *Anesthesia, 36*, 210 – 212.

Classen, W. (1989). Schmerz und Persoenlichkeit: Eine Literaturuebersicht mit besonderer Beruecksichtigung depressiver Syndrome. /Pain and personality: A review of the literature emphasizing depressive syndromes. *Zeitschrift fuer Klinische Psychologie, Psychopathologie und Psychotherapie, 37*, 146-161.

Cobb, S. (1959). Contained hostility in rheumatoid arthritis. *Arthritis and Rheumatology, 2*, 419-425.

Colligan, K. G. (1987). Music therapy and hospice care. *Activities, Adaptation & Aging, 10*, 103-122.

Connant, L. L. (1998). Psychological variables associated with pain perceptions among individuals with chronic spinal cord injury pain. *Journal of Clinical Psychology in Medical Settings, 5*, 71-90.

Cook, W., & Medley, D. (1954). Proposed hostility and pharisiac-virtue scales for the MMPI. *The Journal of Applied Psychology, 38*, 414-418.

Corbishley, M., Hendrickson, R., & Beutler, L. (1990). Behavior, affect, and cognition among psychogenic pain patients in group expressive psychotherapy. *Journal of Pain and Symptom Management, 5*, 241-248.

Cormier, L. E., Katon, W., Russo, J., Hollifield, M., et al (1988). Chest pain with negative cardiac diagnostic studies: Relationship to psychiatric illness. *Journal of Nervous & Mental Disease, 176*, 351-358.

Cornwall, A., & Donderi, D. C. (1988). The effect of experimentally induced anxiety on the experience of pressure pain. *Pain, 35*, 105-113.

Costello, C. G. & Lazarus, A. A. (1972). Depression: Loss of reinforcers or loss of reinforcer effectiveness? *Behavior Therapy, 3*, 240-252.

Couch, J. R., Ziegler, D. K., & Hassanein, R. (1976). Amitriptyline in the prophylaxis of migraine. *Neurology, 26*, 121-127.

Covino, N. A., Dirks, J. F., Fisch, R. I., & Seidel, J. V. (1983). Characteristics of depression of chronically ill medical patients: An elaboration of personality styles. *Psychotherapy & Psychosomatics, 39*, 10-22.

Cox, D., & Thomas, D. (1981). Relationship between headaches and depression. *Headache, 21*, 261-263.

Crisson, J., Keefe, F.J., Wilkins, R. H., Cook, W. A., & Muhlbaier, L. H. (1986). Self-report of depressive symptoms in low back pain patients. *Journal of Clinical Psychology, 42*, 425-430.

Crombez, G., Vlaeyen, J. W. S., Heuts, P. H. T. G., & Lysens, R. (1999). Pain-related fear is more disabling than pain itself: Evidence on the role of pain-related fear in chronic back pain disability. *Pain, 80*, 329-339.

Crook, J., Rideout, E., & Brown, G. (1984). The prevalence of pain complaints in a general population. *Pain, 18,* 299-314.

Crowne, D. P., & Marlowe, D. (1960). A new scale of social desirability independent of psychopathology. *Journal of Consulting Psychology, 24,* 349-354.

Curtiss, G., Kinder, B., Kalichman, S., & Spana, R. (1988). Affective differences among subgroups of chronic pain patients. *Anxiety Research, 1,* 65-73.

Daniels, L. K. (1976). The treatment of acute anxiety and post-operative gingival pain by hypnosis and covert conditioning: A case report. *American Journal of Clinical Hypnosis, 19,* 116-119.

Davey, G. C. (1989). Dental phobias and anxieties: Evidence for conditioning processes in the acquisition and modulation of a learned fear. *Behaviour Research & Therapy, 27,* 51-58.

Davidson. (1994). On emotion, mood, and related affective constructs. In P. Ekman & R. J. Davidson (Eds.), *The Nature of Emotion: Fundamental Questions* (pp. 51-55). New York: Oxford University Press.

Davidson, J., Krishnan, R., France, R. D., & Pelton, S. (1985). Neurovegetative symptoms in chronic pain and depression. *Journal of Affective Disorders, 9,* 213-218.

Davis, C. A. (1992). The effects of music and basic relaxation instruction on pain and anxiety of women undergoing in-office gynecological procedures. *Journal of Music Therapy, 29,* 202-216.

Davis, G. C., Buchsbaum, M. S., Bunney, W. E. (1979). Analgesia to painful stimuli in affective illness. *American Journal of Psychiatry, 136,* 1148-1151.

Deardorff, W. (2001). Minnesota Multiphasic Personality Inventory (MMPI) and Minnesota Multiphasic Personality Inventory -2 (MMPI-2). In R.J. Gatchel (Ed.), *Compendium of outcome intruments for assessment and research of spinal disorders.* LaGrange, IL: North American Spine Society.

Deffenbacher, J. L., Dahlen, E. R., Lynch, R. S., Morris, C. D., & Gowensmith, W. N. (2000). An application of Beck's cognitive therapy to general anger reduction. *Cognitive Therapy & Research*, *24*, 689-697.

DeGood, D. E., Buckelew, S. P., & Tait, R. C. (1985). Cognitive-somatic anxiety response patterning in chronic pain patients and nonpatients. *Journal of Consulting & Clinical Psychology*, *53*, 137-138.

DeGroot, K. I., Boeke, S., van den Berge, H. J., Duivenvoorden, H. J., Bonke, B., & Passchier, J. (1997). Assessing short- and long-term recovery from lumbar surgery with pre-operative biographical, medical and psychological variables. *British Journal of Health Psychology*, *2*, 229-243.

Delaplaine, R., Ifabumuyi, D. I., Merskey, H., & Zarfas, H. (1978). Significance of pain in psychiatric hospital patients. *Pain*, *4*, 361-366.

Delle Chiaie, R., & Teodori, A. (1985). Therapy with tricyclic antidepressants in psychosomatic disorders. *Medicina Psicosomatica, 30*, 251-274.

Dellemijn, P. L. I., & Fields, H. L. (1994). Do benzodiazepines have a role in chronic pain management? *Pain*, *57*, 137-152.

Derogatis, L. R. (1977). SCL-90 administration, scoring and procedures manual. Baltimore, Maryland: Johns Hopkins University Press.

Derogatis, L. R. (1983). The SCL-90-R manual II. Administration, scoring and procedures. Towson, Maryland: Clinical Psychometric Research.

DeVellis, B. M. (1993). Depression in rheumatological diseases. Psychological aspects of rheumatoid disease. *Bailiere's Clinical Rheumatology*, *7*, 241-258.

Diamond, E. (1982). The role of anger and hostility in essential hypertension and coronary heart disease. *Psychological Bulletin*, *92*, 410-433.

Diamond, S. (1964). Depressive headaches. *Headache*, *4*, 255-258.

Dionne, C., & Turcotte, F. (1992). Coping with low-back pain: Remaining disabilities 5 years after multidisciplinary rehabilitation. *Journal of Occupational Rehabilitation, 2*, 73-88.

Dohrenwend, B., Marbach, J., Raphael, K., & Gallagher, R. M. (1999). Why is depression co-morbid with chronic facial pain? A family study test of alternative hypothesis. *Pain, 83*, 183-192.

Dolan, J., Allen, H. A., & Sawyer, H. W. (1982). Relaxation techniques in the reduction of pain, nausea and sleep disturbances for oncology patients: A primer for rehabilitation counselors. *Journal of Applied Rehabilitation Counseling, 13*, 35-39.

Domar, A. D., Noe, J. M., & Benson, H. (1987). The preoperative use of the relaxation response with ambulatory surgery patients. *Journal of Human Stress, 13*, 101-107.

Dorpat, T. L., Anderson, W. F., & Ripley, H. S. (1968). The relationship of physical illness to suicide. In H.L.P. Resnick (Ed.), *Suicidal behaviours: Diagnosis and management* (pp. 209-219). Boston: Little Brown.

Dougher, M. J. (1979). Sensory decision theory analysis of the effects of anxiety and experimental instructions on pain. *Journal of Abnormal Psychology, 88*, 137-144.

Dougher, M. J., Goldstein, D., & Leight, K. A. (1987). Induced anxiety and pain. *Journal of Anxiety Disorders, 1*, 259-264.

Dowhrenwend, B. P., Raphael, K. G., Marbach, J. J., Gallagher, R. M., (1999). Why is depression comorbid with chronic myofascial face pain? A family study test of alternative hypotheses. *Pain, 83*, 183-192.

Dura, J. R., & Beck, S. J. (1988). A comparison of family functioning when mothers have chronic pain. *Pain, 35*, 79-89.

DuRant, R. H., Jay, S., Jerath, R., & Fink, S. (1988). The influence of anxiety and locus of control on adolescents' response to naproxen sodium for mild to moderate pain. *Journal of Adolescent Health Care, 9*, 424-430.

Duthie, A. M. (1976). The use of phenothiazines and tricyclic anti-depressants in the treatment of intractable pain. *Southern Medical Journal, 69*, 246 – 247.

Dworkin, R., & Gitlin, M. J. (1991). Clinical aspects of depression in chronic pain patients. *Clinical Journal of Pain, 7*, 79–94.

Dworkin, R. H, Clark, W. C., & Lipsitz, J. D. (1995). Pain responsivity in major depression and bipolar disorder. *Psychiatry Research, 56*, 173 - 181.

Dworkin, R. H., Hartstein, G., Rosner, H., Walther, R. R. et al (1992). A high-risk method for studying psychosocial antecedents of chronic pain: The prospective investigation of herpes zoster. *Journal of Abnormal Psychology, 101*, 200-205.

Dworkin, S. F., von Korff, M., & LeResche, L. (1990). Multiple pains and psychiatric disturbance: An epidemiologic investigation. *Archives of General Psychiatry, 47*, 239-244.

Eckhardt, C. I., & Deffenbacher, J. L. (1995*). Anger disorders: Definition, diagnosis, and treatment.* Washington, D.C.: Taylor & Francis.

Edwards, L., Pearce, S., Collet, B. J., & Pugh, R. (1992). Selective memory for sensory and affective information in chronic pain and depression. *British Journal of Clinical Psychology, 31*, 239-248.

Ehlert, U., Heim, C., & Hellhammer, D. H., (1999). Chronic pelvic pain as a somatoform disorder. *Psychotherapy and Psychosomatics, 68*, 87-94.

Eifert, G. H. (1992). Cardiophobia: A paradigmatic behavioural model of heart-focused anxiety and non-anginal chest pain. *Behaviour Research & Therapy, 30*, 329-345.

Elias, M. F, et al (1982). A behavioral study of middle-aged chest pain patients: Physical symptom reporting, anxiety, and depression. *Experimental Aging Research, 8* 45-51.

Eller, Lucille Sanzero (1998). Testing a model: Effects of pain on immunity in HIV+ and HIV- participants. *Scholarly Inquiry for Nursing Practice, 12*, 191-214.

Elliott, T. R., & Harkins, S. W. (1992). Emotional distress and the perceived interference of menstruation. *Journal of Psychopathology and Behavioral Assessment, 14*, 293-306.

Ellis, A. (1962). *Reason and emotion in psychotherapy*. New York: Lyle Stewart.

Ellis, A., & Grieger, R. (Eds.), (1986). *Handbook of rational-emotive therapy* (Vols. 1-2). New York: Springer.

Ellis, H. C., & Hunt, R. R. (1993). *Fundamentals of cognitive psychology*. Madison, WI: Brown and Benchmark.

Elton, D., Vagg, P. R., & Stanley, G. V. (1978). Augmentation, reduction and pain experience. *Perceptual & Motor Skills, 47*, 499-502.

Endicott, J., & Spitzer, R. L. (1978). A diagnostic interview: The schedule for Affective Disorders and Schizophrenia. *Archives of General Psychiatry, 35*, 837-844.

Engel, C. C., Von Korff, M., Katon, W. J. (1996). Back pain in primary care: Predictors of high health-care costs. *Pain, 65*, 197-204.

Engel, G. L. (1959). "Psychogenic" pain and the pain prone patient. *American Journal of Medicine, 26*, 899-918.

Engle, E. W., Callahan, L. F., Pincus, T., & Hochberg, M. C. (1990). Learned helplessness in systemic lupus erythematosus: analysis using the Rheumatology Attitudes Index. *Arthritis and Rheumatism, 33*, 281-286.

Estlander, A. M., Takala, E. P., & Verkasalo, M. (1995). Assessment of depression in chronic musculoskeletal pain patients. *Clinical Journal of Pain, 11*, 194-200.

Evans, D. R., & Strangeland, M. (1971). Development of the Reaction Inventory to measure anger. *Psychological Reports, 29*, 412-414.

Evans, W., Gensler, F., Blackwell, B., & Galbrecht, C. (1973). The effects of antidepressant drugs on pain relief and mood in the chronically ill. *Psychosomatics, 14*, 214 – 219.

Eysenck, H. J. (1964). The measurement of personality: A new inventory. *Journal of the Indian Academy of Applied Psychology, 1,* 1-11.

Eysenck, H. J., & Eysenck, S. B. G. (1975). *Manual of the Eysenck Personality Questionnaire.* London: Hodder & Stroughton.

Faravelli, C., Masini, C., & Poli, E. (1979). Headache in depressive syndromes: a clinical study. *Rivista di Patologia Nervosa e Mentale, 100,* 15-27.

Farthing, G.W., Venturino, M., Brown, S. W., & Lazar, J. D. (1997). Internal and external distraction in the control of cold-pressor pain as a function of hypnotizability. *International Journal of Clinical & Experimental Hypnosis, 45,* 433-446.

Fava, G. A., Pilowsky, I., Pierfederici, A., Bernardi, M., & Pathak, D. (1982). Depression and illness behavior in a general hospital: A prevalence study. *Psychotherapy and Psychosomatics, 38,* 141-153.

Faymonville, M.E., Mambourg, P.H., Joris, J., Vrigens, B., Fissette, J., Albert, A., & Lamy, M. (1997). Psychological approaches during conscious sedation. Hypnosis versus stress reducing strategies: A prospective randomized study. *Pain, 73,* 361-367.

Feinmann, C. (1985). Pain relief by antidepressants: Possible modes of action. *Pain, 23,* 1-8.

Feldman, S. I., Downey, G., & Schaffer-Neitz, R. (1999). Pain, negative mood, and perceived support in chronic pain patients: A daily diary study of people with reflex sympathetic dystrophy syndrome. *Journal of Consulting and Clinical Psychology, 67,* 776-785.

Fenton, F. R., Cole, M. G., Engelsmann, F., & Mansouri, I. (1994). Depression in older medical inpatients. *Journal of Geriatric Psychiatry, 9,* 279-284.

Ferguson, E. D. (2000). *Motivation: A biosocial and cognitive integration of motivation and emotion.* New York: Oxford University Press.

Ferguson, R. J., & Ahles, T. A. (1998). Private body consciousness, anxiety and pain symptom reports of chronic pain
patients. *Behaviour Research & Therapy, 36*, 527-535.

Ferguson, S. J., & Cotton, S. (1996). Broken sleep, pain, disability,
social activity, and depressive symptoms in rheumatoid
arthritis. *Australian Journal of Psychology, 48*, 9-14.

Fernandez, E. (1986). A classification system of cognitive coping
strategies for pain. *Pain, 26*, 141-151.

Fernandez, E. (1996). *The Targets and Reasons for Anger in Pain
Sufferers: A Structured Interview*. Unpublished manuscript,
Southern Methodist University.

Fernandez, E. (1998a). Review of the Hamilton Depression In-
ventory. In J. C. Impara & B. S. Plake (Eds.), *The 13th
Mental Measurements Yearbook* (pp.476-477). Lincoln,
NE: Buros Institute of Mental Measurements.

Fernandez, E. (1998b). The role of affect in somatoform and
factitious disorders. *Current Review of Pain, 2*, 109-114.

Fernandez, E. (1999). *Integrating therapeutic techniques: The case
of anger.* The First Mid-Atlantic Conference, Society for
Psychotherapy Research, Baltimore.

Fernandez, E. (2001). *Sequential Integration of Cognitive-
Behavioral and Experiential Techniques for Regulating
Anger.* Workshop conducted at the Annual Conference of
the Society for the Exploration of Psychotherapy
Integration, Santiago, Chile, June 15 2001.

Fernandez, E. (in press). Prevention of anger in children. In T.
Gullotta & M. Bloom (Eds.). *The encyclopedia of primary
prevention and health promotion.* New York: Kluwer
Academic/Plenum Publishers.

Fernandez, E., & Beck, R. (2001). Cognitive-behavioral self-
intervention versus self-monitoring of anger: Effects on
anger frequency, duration, and intensity. *Behavioural and
Cognitive Psychotherapy, 29*, 345-356.

Fernandez, E., & Boyle, G. J. (2002). Affective and evaluative descriptors of pain in the McGill Pain Questionnaire:

Reduction and reorganization. *The Journal of Pain*, *3*, 70-77.

Fernandez, E., Clark, T. S., & Rudick-Davis, D. (1999). A framework for conceptualization and assessment of affective disturbance in pain. In A.R. Block, E.F. Kremer, & E. Fernandez (Eds.), *Handbook of Pain Syndromes: Biopsychosocial perspectives* (pp. 123-147). Mahwah, NJ: Erlbaum.

Fernandez, E., & McDowell, J. J. (1995). Response-reinforcement relationships in chronic pain syndrome: Applicability of Herrnstein's law. *Behaviour Research and Therapy*, *33*, 855-863.

Fernandez, E., & Milburn, T. E. (1994). Sensory and affective predictors of overall pain, and emotions associated with affective pain, *The Clinical Journal of Pain*, *10*, 3-9.

Fernandez, E., & Scott, S. (manuscript in submission). Anger in chemically-dependent inpatients: Treatment outcome and gender differences.

Fernandez, E., & Towery, S. (1996). A parsimonious set of verbal descriptors of pain sensation derived from the McGill Pain Questionnaire. *Pain*, *66*, 31-37.

Fernandez, E., & Turk, D. C. (1992). Sensory and affective components of pain: Separation and synthesis. *Psychological Bulletin*, *112*, 205-217.

Fernandez, E., & Turk, D. C. (1993). Anger in chronic pain: A neglected target of attention. *American Pain Society Bulletin*, *3*, 5-7.

Fernandez, E., & Turk, D. C. (1994). Demand characteristics underlying differential ratings of sensory versus affective components of pain. *Journal of Behavioral Medicine*, *17*, 375-389.

Fernandez, E., & Turk, D. C. (1995). The scope and significance of anger in the experience of chronic pain. *Pain*, *61*, 165-175.

Feshbach, S. (1986). Reconceptualizations of anger: Some research perspectives. *Journal of Social and Clinical Psychology*, *4*, 123-132.

Feuerstein, M. (1986). *Ambulatory monitoring of paraspinal skeletal muscle, autonomic and mood-pain interaction in chronic low back pain*. Paper presented at the Seventh Annual Meeting of the Society of Behavioral Medicine, San Francisco.

Feuerstein, M., Bortolussi, L., Houle, M., & Labbe, E. (1983). Stress, temporal artery activity, and pain in migraine headache: A prospective analysis. *Headache*, *23*, 296-304.

Field, T., Hernandez-Reif, M., Seligman, S., Krasnegor, J., Sunshine, W., Rivas-Chacon, R., Schanberg, S., & Kuhn, C. (1997). Juvenile rheumatoid arthritis: Benefits from massage therapy. *Journal of Pediatric Psychology*, *22*, 607-617.

Fields, H. (1991). Depression and pain: A neurobiological model. *Neuropsychiatry, Neuropsychology, & Behavioral Neurology*, *4*, 83-92.

Fifield, Judith; Reisine, Susan T.; Grady, Kathleen E. (1991). Work disability and the experience of pain and depression in rheumatoid arthritis. *Social Science & Medicine*, *33*, 579-585.

Fishbain, D. A., Cutler, R., Rosomoff, H. L., & Rosomoff, R. S. (1997). Chronic pain-associated depression: Antecedent or consequence of chronic pain? A review. *Clinical Journal of Pain*, *13*, 116-137.

Fishbain, D. A., Goldberg, M., Meagher, B. R., & Steele, R. (1986). Male and female chronic pain categorized by DSM-III psychiatric diagnostic criteria. *Pain*, *26*, 181-197.

Flor, H., & Turk, D. C. (1989). Psychophysiology of chronic pain: Do chronic pain patients exhibit symptom-specific psychophysiological responses? *Psychological Bulletin*, *105*, 215-259.

Flor, H., Birbaumer, N., Schugens, M. M., & Lutzenberger, W. (1992). Symptom-specific psychophysiological responses in chronic pain patients. *Psychophysiology, 29,* 452-460.

Folkins, C. H., & Sime, W. E. (1981). Physical fitness training and mental health. *American Psychologist, 36,* 373-389.

Ford, C. V. (1995). Dimensions of somatization and hypochondriasis. Special issue: Malingering and conversion reactions. *Neurologic Clinics, 13,* 241-253.

Fordyce, W. E. (1976). *Behavioral methods for chronic pain and illness.* St. Louis: Mosby.

Fowler-Kerry, S., & Lander, J. (1991). Assessment of sex differences in children's and adolescents' self-reported pain from venipuncture. *Journal of Pediatric Psychology, 16,* 783-793.

France, R. D. (1987). The future for antidepressants: Treatment of pain. *Psychopathology, 20,* 99-113.

France, R. D., Houpt, J. L., & Ellinwood, E. H. (1984). Therapeutic effects of antidepressants in chronic pain. *General Hospital Psychiatry, 6,* 55-63.

Frances, A. & Kroll, J. (1989). Ongoing treatment of a Hmong widow who suffers from pain and depression. *Hospital and Community Psychiatry, 40,* 691-693.

Franz, C., Paul, R., Bautz, M., Choroba, B., & Hildebrandt, J. (1986). Psychosomatic aspects of chronic pain: A new way of description based on MMPI item analysis. *Pain, 26,* 33-43.

Freeman, C., Calsyn, D., & Louks, J. (1976). The use of the Minnesota Multiphasic Personality Inventory with low back pain patients. *Journal of Clinical Psychology, 32,* 294-298.

Freemont, J., & Craighead, L. W. (1987). Aerobic exercise and cognitive therapy in the treatment of dysphoric moods. *Cognitive Therapy and Research, 11,* 241-251.

French, A. P., & Tupin, J. P. (1974). Therapeutic application of a simple relaxation method. *American Journal of Psychotherapy, 28,* 282-287.

Freud, S. (1937). Analysis terminable and interminable. Standard Edition of the Complete Works of Sigmund Freud, 23, 216-253. London: Hogarth Press, 1964.

Freud, S. (1915). *Instincts and their vicissitudes, collected papers (Vol. 4, pp. 60-83)*. New York: Basic Books.

Freud, S. (1934). Mourning and melancholia (1917). In S. Freud *Collected Papers, Vol.4* London: Hogarth Press.

Freud, S. (1940). An outline of psycho-analysis. Standard Edition of the Complete Works of Sigmund Freud, 23, 144-207. London: Hogarth Press, 1964.

Frid, M., & Singer, G. (1979). Hypnotic analgesia in conditions of stress is partially reversed by naloxone. *Psychopharmacology, 63*, 211-215.

Fried, R. (1993). *The psychology and physiology of breathing in behavioral medicine, clinical psychology, and psychiatry.* New York: Plenum Press.

Friedman, A. S. (1970). Hostility factors and clinical improvement in depressed patients. *Archives in General Psychiatry, 23*, 523.

Friedman, H. S. (Ed.), (1992). *Hostility, coping and health.* Washington, DC: American Psychological Association.

Frijda, N. H. (1986). *The emotions.* Cambridge: Cambridge University Press.

Frijda, N. H., Kuipers, P., & ter Schure, E. (1989). Relations among emotions, appraisal, and emotional action readiness. *Journal of Personality and Social Psychology, 57*, 212-228.

Fuqua, D. R., Leonard, E., Masters, M. A., Smith, R. J., Campbell, J. L,, & Fischer, P.C. (1991). A structural analysis of the State-Trait Anger Expression Inventory (STAXI). *Educational and Psychological Measurement, 51*, 439-446.

Gabert-Varga, U., Schmid, M., & Revenstorf, D. Einstreutechnik und therapeutische Anekdoten zur Behandlung akuter Schmerzen. Eine empirische Untersuchung. (1991). Interspersal techniques and therapeutic anecdotes in the treatment of acute pain: An empirical study. *Experimentelle und Klinische Hypnose, 7,* 109-146.

Gagliano, M. E. (1988). A literature review on the efficacy of video in patient education. *Journal of Medical Education, 63,* 785-792.

Gagliese, L., & Melzack, R. (1997). Chronic pain in elderly people. *Pain, 70,* 3-14.

Gallagher, R.M., Moore, P., & Chernoff, I. (1995a). The reliability of depression diagnosis in chronic low back pain: a pilot study. *General Hospital Psychiatry, 17,* 399-413.

Gamsa, A. (1990). Is emotional disturbance a precipitator or a consequence of chronic pain? *Pain, 42,* 183-195.

Garron, D. C., & Leavitt, F. (1979). Demographic and affective covariates of pain. *Psychosomatic Medicine, 41,* 525-534.

Garron, D. C., & Leavitt, F., (1983). Chronic low-back pain and depression. *Journal of Clinical Psychology, 39,* 486-493.

Gaskin, M. E., Green, A. F., Robinson, M. E., & Geisser M. E. (1992). Negative affect and the experience of pain. *Journal of Psychosomatic Research, 36,* 707 - 713.

Gatchel, R. J. (1996). Psychological disorders and chronic pain: Cause-and-effect relationships. In R. J. Gatchel & D. C. Turk (Eds.), *Psychological approaches to pain management: A practitioner's handbook* (pp. 33-52). New York: Guilford Press.

Gatchel, R. J. & Weisberg, J. N. (Eds.), (2000). *Personality characteristics of patients with pain.* Washington, DC, US: American Psychological Association.

Gay, C., & Boureau, F. (1989). Douleur et depression. /Pain and depression. *Confrontations Psychiatriques, Spec. Issue,* 120-131.

Geisser, M. E., Roth, R. S., Bachman, J. E., & Eckert, T. A. (1996). The relationship between symptoms of post-traumatic stress disorder and pain, affective disturbance and disability among patients. with accident and non-accident related pain. *Pain, 66,* 207-214.

Genuis, M. L. (1995). The use of hypnosis in helping cancer patients control anxiety, pain, and emesis: A review of recent empirical studies. *American Journal of Clinical Hypnosis, 37,* 316-325.

Georganda, E. (1990). The impact of thalassemia on body image, self-image, and self-esteem. *Annals of the New York Academy of Sciences, 612,* 466-472.

Gershon, E. S., Cromer, M., & Klerman, G. L. (1968). Hostility and depression. *Psychiatry, 31,* 224-235.

Getka, E. J., Glass, C. R. (1992). Behavioral and cognitive-behavioral approaches to the reduction of dental anxiety. *Behavior Therapy, 23,* 433-448.

Getto, C. J., Sorkness, C. A., & Howell, T. (1987). Antidepressants and chronic nonmalignant pain: A review. *Journal of Pain and Symptom Management, 2,* 9-18.

Gibson, J. J. (1979). *The ecological approach to visual perception.* Boston: Houghton Mifflin.

Glover, J., Dibble, S.L., Dodd, M.J., Miaskkowski, C., (1995). Mood states of oncology outpatients: Does pain make a difference? *Journal of Pain and Symptom Management, 10,* 120-128.

Gomersall, J. D., & Stuart, A. (1973). Amitriptyline in migraine prophylaxis. *Journal of Neurology, Neurosurgery, and Psychiatry, 36,* 684 – 690.

Gonzales, G. R. (1995). Central pain: Diagnosis and treatment strategies. *Neurology, 45,* S11-S16.

Gonzales, J. R., Lee, R. L., Sewell, R. P. E., & Spencer, P. S. J. (1980). Antidepressants and pain. A review of some human and animal studies. *Roy. Soc. Med. Suppl., 25,* 59-69.

Goodyer, I., & Cooper, P.J. (1993). A coomunity study of depression in adolescent girls: II. The clinical features of identified disorder. *British Journal of Psychiatry, 163,* 374-380.

Gotlib, I. H. (1984). Depression and general psychopathology in university students. *Journal of Abnormal Psychology, 93,* 19-30.

Gracely, R. H. (1992). Evaluation of multi-dimensional pain scales. *Pain, 48,* 297-300.

Graulich, P., Segers, M. J., Mertens, C., Vastesaeger, M. (1975). Anxiety, depression, and angina: Epidemiological data. *Journal of Psychosomatic Research, 19,* 55-67.

Graver, V., Ljunggren, A. E., Malt, U. F., Loeb, M., et al (1995). Can psychological traits predict the outcome of lumbar disc surgery when anamnestic and physiological risk factors are controlled for? Results of a prospective cohort study. *Journal of Psychosomatic Research, 39,* 465-476.

Greenberg, L. S., & Safran, J. D. (1990). In R. Plutchik & H. Kellerman (Eds.), *Emotion theory research and experience volume 5: Emotion, psychopathology, and psychotherapy.* San Diego: Academic Press.

Gringas, M. (1976). A clinical trial of tofranil in rheumatic pain in general practice. *Journal of Internal Med. Res., 4,* 41-49.

Gross, R. T., Collins, F. L. (1981). On the relationship between anxiety and pain: A methodological confounding. *Clinical Psychology Review, 1,* 375-386.

Gupta, M. A. (1986). Is chronic pain a variant of depressive illness? A critical review. *Canadian Journal of Psychiatry, 31,* 241-248.

Haley, W. E., Turner, J. A., & Romano, J. M. (1985). Depression in chronic pain patients: Relation to pain, activity, and sex differences. *Pain, 23,* 337-343.

Hall, K. R. L., & Stride, E. (1954). The varying response to pain in psychiatric disorders: a study in abnormal psychology. *British Journal of Medical Psychology, 27,* 48-60.

Halper, J. P., & Mann, J. J. (1988). Cardiovascular effects of antidepressant medications. *British Journal of Psychiatry, 153,* 87-98.

Hameroff, S. R., Cork, R. C., Scherer, K., Crago, B. R., Neuman, C., & Womble Jr., Davis, T. P. (1982). Doxepin effects on chronic pain, depression and plasma opoids. *Journal of Clinical Psychiatry, 43*, 22 – 26.

Hamilton, M. (1960). A rating scale for depression. *Journal of Neurology, Neurosurgery and Psychiatry, 23*, 56-62.

Hamilton, M. (1967). Development of a rating scale for primary depressive illness. *British Journal of Social and Clinical Psychology, 6*, 278-296.

Hanks, G. W. (1981). Antidepressants in postherpetic neuralgia: A double-blind study to investigate efficacy and possible mode of action (abstract). *Pain Suppl. 1*, S96.

Hardy, J. D., & Smith, T. W. (1988). Cynical hostility and vulnerability to disease: Social support, life stress, and physiological response to conflict. *Health Psychology, 7*, 447-459.

Hardy, J. D., Wolff, H. G., & Goodell, H. (1952). *Pain sensations and reactions*. Baltimore: Williams and Wilkins.

Hatch, J., Schoenfeld, L., Boutros N.N., Seleshi, E., Moore, P., & Cyr-Provost, M. (1991). Anger and hostility in tension-type headache. *Headache, 31*, 302-304.

Hathaway, S. R., & McKinley, J. C. (1943). *The Minnesota Multiphasic Personality Schedule*. Minneapolis, MN: University of Minnesota Press.

Hawkins, P. J., Liossi, C., Ewart, B. W., Hatira, P., Kosmidis, V. H. (1998). Hypnosis in the alleviation of procedure related pain and distress in paediatric oncology patients. *Contemporary Hypnosis, 15*, 199-207.

Hawley, D. J., & Wolfe, F. (1988). Anxiety and depression in patients with rheumatoid arthritis: A prospective study of 400 patients. *Journal of Rheumatology, 15*, 932-941.

Haythornthwaite, J. A., Sieber, W. J., & Kerns, R. D. (1991). Depression and the chronic pain experience. *Pain, 46*, 177-184.

Heath, R. G. (1986). The neural substrate for emotion. In R. Plutchik & H. Kellerman (Eds.), *Emotion: Theory, re-*

search and experience: Vol. 3. Biological foundations of emotion (pp. 37-60). New York: Academic Press.

Hedlund, J. L., & Vieweg, B. W. (1981). Structured psychiatric interviews: A comparative review. *Journal of Operational Psychiatry, 12,* 39-67.

Heider, F. (1958). *The psychology of interpersonal relations.* New York: Wiley.

Heim, H. M., & Oei, T. P. (1993). Comparison of prostate cancer patients with and without pain. *Pain, 53,* 159-162.

Heitkemper, T., Layne, C., Sullivan, D. M. (1993). Brief treatment of children's dental pain and anxiety. *Perceptual & Motor Skills, 76,* 192-194.

Helmes, E., & Reddon, J. R. (1993). A perspective on developments in assessing psychopathology: a critical review of the MMPI and MMPI-2. *Psychological Bulletin, 113,* 453-471.

Hendler, N. (1984). Depression caused by chronic pain. *Journal of Clinical Psychiatry, 45,* 30-38.

Hilgard, E. R. (1977). Divided consciousness: Multiple controls in human thought and action. New York: Wiley.

Hilgard, E. R., & Hilgard, J. R. (1975). Hypnosis in the relief of pain. Los Altos, CA: Kaufman.

Hill, H. E., Flanary, H. G., Kornetsky, C. H., & Wikler, A. (1952). Effects of anxiety and morphine on discrimination of intensities of painful stimuli. *Journal of Clinical Investigation, 31,* 473-480.

Himell, K. (1981). Genital herpes: The need for counseling. *Journal of Gynecological Nursing, 10,* 446-450.

Hirt, M., Kurtz, R., & Ross, W. D. (1967). The relationship between dysmennorhea and select personality variables. *Psychosomatics, 8,* 350-353.

Hitchcock, L. S., Ferrell, B. R., & McCaffery, M. (1994). The experience of chronic nonmalignant pain. *Journal of Pain and Symptom Management, 9,* 312-318.

Hodges, K., Kline, J. J., Barbero, G., & Woodruff, C. (1985). Anxiety in children with recurrent abdominal pain and their parents. *Psychosomatics, 26,* 859-866.

Hodgkiss, A. D., Sufraz, R., & Watson, J. P. (1994). Psychiatric morbidity and illness behaviour in women with chronic pelvic pain. *Journal of Psychosomatic Research, 38,* 3-9.

Hoeper, E. W., Nyczi, G. R., Cleary, P. D., & Goldberg, I. D. (1979). Estimated prevalence of RDC mental disorder in primary care. *International Journal of Mental Health, 8,* 6-15.

Holmes, T. H., & Rahe, R. H. (1967). The Social Readjustment Rating Scale. *Journal of Psychosomatic Research, 11,* 213-218.

Holroyd, K. A., Talbot, F., Holm, J. E., Pingel, J. D., Lake, A. E., & Saper, J. R. (1996). Asssessing the dimensions of pain: a multitrait-multimethod evaluation of seven measures. *Pain, 67,* 259-265.

Horvath, A. O., & Symonds, B. D. (1991). Relations between working alliance and outcome in psychotherapy: A meta-analysis. *Journal of Consulting and Clinical Psychology, 38,* 139-149.

Houston, B. K., & Kelley, K. E. (1989). Hostility in employed women: Relation to work and marital experiences, social support, stress, and anger expression. *Personality and Social Psychology Bulletin, 15,* 175-182.

Ingram, R. E., Atkinson, J. H., Slater, M. A., & Saccuzzo, D. P. (1990). Negative and positive cognition in depressed and nondepressed chronic-pain patients. *Health Psychology, 9,* 300-314.

Ingram, R. E., Slater, M. A., Atkinson, J. H., & Scott, W. (1990). Positive automatic cognition in major affective disorder. *Psychological Assessment, 2,* 209-211.

International Association for the Study of Pain (1986). Classification of chronic pain: Descriptions of chronic pain syndromes and definitions of pain terms. *Pain* (Suppl. 3), S1-S226.

Iovchuk, N. M. (1985-1986). Endogenous depressions in children. *Soviet Neurology & Psychiatry, 18,* 61-70.

Izard, C. E. (1977). *Human emotions.* New York: Plenum Press.

Izard, C. E. (1993). Four systems for emotion activation: cognitive and noncognitive processes. *Psychological Review, 100,* 68-90.

Jacobson, E. (1938). Progressive relaxation (2nd edition). Chicago: University of Chicago Press.

James, W. (1890). *The principles of psychology, Vols. 1 and 2.* New York: Henry Holt.

Janssen, S. A., & Arntz, A. (1966). Anxiety and pain: Attentional and endorphinergic influences. *Pain, 66,* 145-150.

Janssen, S. A., & Arntz, A. (1999). No interactive effects of naltrexone and benzodiazepines on pain during phobic fear. *Behaviour Research & Therapy, 37,* 77-86.

Janssen, S. A., & Arntz, A. (1997). Maastricht U, Dept of Medical Psychology, Maastricht, Netherlands No evidence for opioid-mediated analgesia induced by phobic fear. *Behaviour Research & Therapy, 35,* 823-830.

Jenkins, D. G., Ebbutt, A. F., & Evans, C. D. (1976). Tofranil in the treatment of low back pain. *Journal of Internal Medicine Research, 4,* 28 – 40.

Jennings, B. M., & Sherman, R. A. (1987). Anxiety, locus of control, and satisfaction in patients undergoing ambulatory surgery. *Military Medicine, 152,* 206-208.

Jensen, J. (1988). Pain in non-psychotic psychiatric patients: Life events, symptomatology and personality traits. *Acta Psychiatrica Scandinavica, 78,* 201-207.

Jevne, R. (1990). Looking back to look ahead: A retrospective study of referrals to a cancer counselling service. *International Journal for the Advancement of Counseling, 13,* 61-72.

Johnson, J. E., Leventhal, H., & Dabbs, J. M. (1971). Contribution of emotional and instrumental response processes in adaptation to surgery. *Journal of Personality & Social Psychology, 20,* 55-64.

Jones, L. P. (1985). Anxiety, as experienced by chronic pain patients. *Journal of Religion & Health, 24,* 209-217.

Joreskog, K. G. (1978). Structural analysis of covariance and correlation matrices. *Psychometrika, 43*, 443-477.

Joreskog, K. G., & Sorbom, D. (1985). *LISREL-VI: Analysis of linear structural relationships maximum likelihood, instrumental variables and least squares methods*. Department of Statistics, University of Uppsala, Sweden.

Joukamaa, M. (1994). Depression and back pain. *Acta Psychiatrica Scandinavica, 89*, 83-86.

Joyce, P. R., Bushnell, J. A., Walshe, J. W., & Morton, J. B. (1986). Abnormal illness behaviour and anxiety in acute non-organic abdominal pain. *British Journal of Psychiatry, 149*, 57-62.

Karno, J., & Hoffman, R. (1974). The pseudoanergic syndrome. In A. Kiev (Ed.) *Somatic Manifestations of Depressive Disorders*, Amsterdam, Exerpta Medica, 55-85.

Kashani, J., Frank, R., Kashani, S., Wonerlich, S., & Reid, J. (1983). Depression among amputees. *Journal of Clinical Psychiatry, 44*, 256-258.

Kathol, R., Katon, W., Smith, G. R., Petty, F. et al, (1994). Guidelines for the diagnosis and treatment of depression for primary care physicians: Implications for consultation-liasion psychiatrists. *Psychosomatics, 35*, 1-12.

Katon, W., & Sullivan, M. D. (1990). Depression and chronic medical illness. *Journal of Clinical Psychiatry, 51*, 3-11.

Katon, W., Berg, A. O., & Robins, A. J.(1986). Depression: medical utilization and somatization. *Western Journal of Medicine, 144*, 564-568.

Katon, W., Egan, K., & Miller, D. (1985). Chronic pain: Lifetime psychiatric diagnoses and family history. *American Journal of Psychiatry, 142*, 1156-1160.

Katon, W., von Korff, M., Lin, E., Bush, T., Ornel, J., & Lipscomb, P. (1990). Distressed high utilizers of medical care: DSM-III--R diagnoses and treatment needs. *General Hospital Psychiatry, 12*, 355-362.

Kaye, J. M., & Schindler, B. A. (1990). Hypnosis on a consultation liaison service. *General Hospital Psychiatry, 12*, 379-383.

Keefe, F. J., Beaupre, P. M., & Gil, K. M. (1996). Group therapy for patients with chronic pain. In R. J. Gatchel & D. C. Turk (Eds). *Psychological approaches to pain management: A practitioner's handbook.* (pp. 259-282). New York: The Guilford Press.

Keefe, F.J; et al (1986). Depression, pain, and pain behavior. *Journal of Consulting & Clinical Psychology, 54*, 665-669.

Keller, L. S., & Butcher, J. N. (1991). *Assessment of chronic pain patients with the MMPI-2.* Minneapolis, MN: University of Minnesota Press.

Kellerman, J., Zeltzer, L., Ellenberg, L., & Dash, J. (1983). Adolescents with cancer: Hypnosis for the reduction of the acute pain and anxiety associated with medical procedures. *Journal of Adolescent Health Care, 4*, 85-90.

Kerns, R. D., & Haythornthwaite, J. A. (1988). Depression among chronic pain patients: Cognitive-behavioral analysis and effect on rehabilitation outcome. *Journal of Consulting and Clinical Psychology, 56*, 870 - 876.

Kerns, R. D., Haythornthwaite, J., Rosenberg, R., Southwick, S., Giller, E. L., & Jacob, M. C. (1991a). The pain behavior checklist (PBCL): Factor structure and psychometric properties. *Journal of Behavioral Medicine, 14*, 155-167.

Kerns, R. D., Rosenberg, R., & Jacob, M. C. (1991b). *Anger expression and chronic pain.* Paper presented at the Tenth Annual Scientific Meeting of the American Pain Society.

Kerns, R. D., Rosenberg, R., & Jacob, M. C. (1994). Anger expression and chronic pain. *Journal of Behavioral Medicine, 17*, 57-67.

Kerns, R. D., Turk, D. C., & Rudy, T. E. (1985). The West Haven-Yale Multidimensional Pain Inventory (WHYMPI). *Pain, 23*, 345-356.

Kessler, R. C., McGonagle, K. A., Zhao, S. et al. (1994). Lifetime and 12-month prevalence of DSM-III-R psychiatric disorders in the United States. *Archives of General Psychiatry, 51*, 8-19.

Kessler, R. C., McGonagle, K. A., Zhao, S., & Nelson, C. B. (1994). Lifetime and 12-month prevalence of DSM-III--R psychiatric disorders in the United States: Results from the National Comorbidity Study. *Archives of General Psychiatry, 51*, 8-19.

Khatami, M., & Rush, A. (1982). John A one year follow-up of the multimodal treatment for chronic pain. *Pain, 14*, 45-52.

Kinder, B., Curtiss, G., & Kalichman, S. (1986). Anxiety and anger as predictors of MMPI elevations in chronic pain patients. *Journal of Personality Assessment, 50*, 651-661.

Kinder, B. N., & Curtiss, G. (1988). Assessment of anxiety, depression, and anger in chronic pain patients: Conceptual and methodological issues. In C.D. Spielberger & J. N. Butcher (Eds.), *Advances in Personality Assessment*, (pp.161-173). Hillsdale, N. J.: Erlbaum.

King, S. A. (1995). Review: DSM-IV and pain. *Clinical Journal of Pain, 11,* 171-176.

Kirsch, I. & Sapirstein, G. (1999). Listening to Prozac but hearing placebo: A meta-analysis of antidepresant medication. In I. Kirch (Ed.), *How expectancies shape experience* . Washington D. C.: American Psychological Association.

Klusman, L.E. (1975). Reduction of pain in childbirth by the alleviation of anxiety during pregnancy. *Journal of Consulting & Clinical Psychology, 43*, 162-165.

Knights, E. B., & Folstein, M. F. (1975). Unsuspected emotional and cognitive disturbance in medical patients. *Annals of Internal Medicine, 87*, 723-724.

Koenig, H., Shelp, F., Goli, V., & Cohen, H. (1989). Survival and health care utilization in elderly medical inpatients with major depression. *Journal of the American Geristrics Society, 37*, 599-606.

Kohler, T., & Haimerl, C. (1990). Daily stress as a trigger of migraine attacks: Results of thirteen single-subject studies.

Journal of Consulting and Clinical Psychology, 58, 870-872.

Kondas, O., & Scetnicka, B. (1972). Systematic desensitization as a method of preparation for childbirth. *Journal of Behavior Therapy & Experimental Psychiatry, 3,* 51-54.

Kori, S. H., Miller, R. P., & Todd, D. D. (1990). Kinisophobia: a new view of chronic pain behavior. *Pain Management, January/February,* 35-43.

Kornetsky, C. (1954). Effects of anxiety and morphine on the anticipation and perception of painful radiant thermal stimuli. *Journal of Comparative & Physiological Psychology, 47,* 130-132.

Krag, N. J., Norregaard, J., Larsen, J. K., Danneskiold-Samsoe, B. (1994). A blinded, controlled evaluation of anxiety and depressive symptoms in patients with fibromyalgia, as measured by standardized psychometric interview scales. *Acta Psychiatrica Scandinavica, 89,* 370-375.

Kramlinger, K. G., Swanson, D. W., & Maruta, T. (1983). Are patients with chronic pain depressed? *American Journal of Psychiatry, 140,* 747-749.

Kreitler, S., Carasso, R., & Kreitler, H. Cognitive styles and personality traits as predictors of response to therapy in pain patients. *Personality & Individual Differences, 10,* 313-322.

Krishnan, K. R., France, R. D., Pelton, S., McCann, U. D., Davidson, J., & Urban, B. J. (1985). Chronic pain and depression: II. Symptoms of anxiety in chronic low back pain patients and their relationship to subtypes of depression. *Pain, 22,* 289-294.

Kristjansdottir, G. K. (1997). The relationships between pains and various discomforts in schoolchildren. *Childhood, 4,* 491-504.

Krug, S. E., & Laughlin, J. E. (1976). Handbook for the IPAT Depression Scale. Champaign, Illinois: Institute for Personality and Ability Testing.

Kuch, K., Cox, B. J., Evans, R. J., Watson, P. C., et al (1993). To what extent do anxiety and depression interact with chronic pain? *Canadian Journal of Psychiatry, 38*, 36-38.

Kurtze, N., Gundersen, K. T., & Svebak, S. (1998). The role of anxiety and depression in fatigue and patterns of pain among subgroups of fibromyalgia patients. *British Journal of Medical Psychology, 71*, 185-194.

Kutner, N. G., Fair, P. L., & Kutner, M. H. (1985). Assessing depression and anxiety in chronic dialysis patients. *Journal of Psychosomatic Research, 29*, 23-31.

Kuttner, L. (1988). Favorite stories: A hypnotic pain-reduction technique for children in acute pain. *American Journal of Clinical Hypnosis, 30*, 289-295.

Kuttner, L. (1989). Management of young children's acute pain and anxiety during invasive medical procedures. *Pediatrician, 16*, 39-44.

Kuttner, L., Bowman, M., & Teasdale, M. (1988). Psychological treatment of distress, pain, and anxiety for young children with cancer. *Journal of Developmental & Behavioral Pediatrics, 9*, 374-381.

Lambert, S. A. (1996). The effects of hypnosis/guided imagery on the postoperative course of children. *Journal of Developmental & Behavioral Pediatrics, 17*, 307-310.

Lance, J. W., & Curran, D. A. (1964). Treatment of chronic tension headache. *Lancet 1*, 1236 – 1239.

Lander, J., Hodgins, M., & Fowler-Kerry, S. (1992). Children's pain predictions and memories. *Behaviour Research & Therapy, 30*, 117-124.

Lane, C., & Hobfoll, S. E. (1992). How loss affects anger and alienates potential supporters. *Journal of Consulting and Clinical Psychology, 60*, 935-942.

Large, R. G. (1982). The psychiatry of chronic pain. *Stress, 3*, 8-14.

Large, R.G. (1986). DSM-III diagnoses in chronic pain: Confusion or clarity? *Journal of Nervous & Mental Disease, 174,* 295-303.

Large, R. G. (1980). The psychiatrist and the chronic pain patient: 172 antidotes. *Pain, 9,* 253 - 263.

Large, R. G. (1986). DSM-III diagnoses in chronic pain: Confusion or clarity? *Journal of Nervous & Mental Disease, 174,* 295-303.

Larsen, D. K., Taylor, S., Asmundson, G. J. G. (1997). Exploratory factor analysis of the pain anxiety symptoms scale in patients with chronic pain complaints. *Pain, 69,* 27-34.

Latimer, P. R. (1983). Irritable bowel syndrome. *Psychosomatics, 24,* 205-218.

Lautenbacher, S., & Krieg, J. C. (1994). Pain perception in psychiatric disorders: A review of the literature. *Journal of Psychiatric Research, 28,* 109-122.

Lautenbacher, S., Roscher, S., Strian, D., Fassbender, K. et al. (1994). Pain perception in depression: Relationships to symptomatology and naloxone-sensitive mechanisms. *Psychosomatic Medicine, 56,* 345-352.

Lazarus, R. S. (1984). On the primacy of cognition. *American Psychologist, 39,* 124-129.

Lazarus, R. S. (1991). Cognition and motivation in emotion. *American Psychologist, 46,* 352-367.

Lazarus, R. S. (1991). Progress on a cognitive-motivational-relational theory of emotion. *American Psychologist, 46,* 819-834.

LeBaron, S., & Zelter, L. (1984). Assessment of acute pain and anxiety in children and adolescents by self-reports, observer reports, and a behavior checklist. *Journal of Consulting & Clinical Psychology, 52,* 729-738.

LeDoux, J. E. (1987). Emotion. In F. Plum (Ed.), *Handbook of physiology: Sec 1. The nervous system: Vol. 5. Higher funtions of the brain* (pp. 419-459). Bethesda, MD: American Psychological Society.

Lee, H. B., Cheung, F. M., Man, H. M., & Hsu, S. Y. (1992). Psychological characteristics of Chinese low back pain patients: An exploratory study. *Psychology & Health, 6,* 119-128.

Lee, J., Giles, K, & Drummond, P. D. (1993). Psychological disturbances and an exaggerated response to pain in patients with whiplash injury. *Journal of Psychosomatic Research, 37,* 105-110.

Lefebvre, M. F. (1981). Cognitive distortion and cognitive errors in depressed psychiatric and low back pain patients. *Journal of Consulting and Clinical Psychology, 49,* 517-525.

Leiker, M., & Hailey, B. (1988). A link between hostility and disease: Poor health habits? *Behavioral Science, 14,* 129-133.

Lesse, S. (1962). Psychotherapy in combination with anti-depressant drugs. American *Journal of Psychotherapy, 16,* 407 - 423.

Lesse, S. (1974). Depression masked by acting-out behavior patterns. *American Journal of Psychotherapy, 28,* 352-361.

Lesse, S. (1983). The masked depression syndrome: Results of a seventeen-year clinical study. *American Journal of Psychotherapy, 37,* 456-475.

Leu, S. J., & Wang, R. H. (1975). Increased analgesia and alterations in distribution and metabolism of methadone and desipramine in the rat. *Journal of Pharmacological Experimental Therapy, 195,* 94-104.

Levenson, J. L., Hamer, R. M., Silverman, J. L., & Rossiter, L. F. (1986-1987). Psychopathology in medical inpatients and its relationship to length of hospital stay: A pilot study. *International Journal of Psychiatry in Medicine, 16,* 231-236.

Leventhal, E. A., & Prochaska, T. R. (1986). Age, symptom interpretation and health behavior. *Journal of the American Gerontological Society, 34,* 183-191.

Levor, R. M., Cohen, M. J., Naliboff, B. D., & McArthur, D. (1986). Psychosocial precursors and correlates of migraine headache. *Journal of Consulting & Clinical Psychology, 54,* 347-353.

Lewinsohn, P. M., Sullivan, J. M., & Grosscup, S. J. (1980). Changing reinforcing events: An approach to the treatment of depression. *Psychotherapy: Theory, Research and Practice, 17,* 322-334.

Lilienfield, A. M., & Lilienfield, D. E. (1980). Foundations of epidemiology. New York: Oxford University Press.

Lindsay, P. G., & Wyckoff, M. (1981). The depression-pain syndrome and its response to antidepressants. *Psychosomatics, 22,* 571-177.

Linton, S. J., & Goetestam, K. G. (1985). Relations between pain, anxiety, mood and muscle tension in chronic pain patients: A correlation study. *Psychotherapy & Psychosomatics, 43,* 90-95.

Liossi, C., & Hatira, P. (1999). Clinical hypnosis versus cognitive behavioral training for pain management with pediatric cancer patients undergoing bone marrow aspirations. *International Journal of Clinical & Experimental Hypnosis, 47,* 104-116.

Lipowski, Z. J. (1990a). Chronic idiopathic pain syndrome. *Annals of Medicine, 22,* 213-217.

Lipowski, Z. J. (1990b). Somatization and depression. *Psychosomatics, 31,* 13-21.

Litt, M. D. (1996). A model of pain and anxiety associated with acute stressors: Distress in dental procedures. *Behaviour Research & Therapy, 34,* 459-476.

Litt, M. D., Cooney, N. L., & Morse, P. (1998). Ecological momentary assessment (EMA) with treated alcoholics: Methodological problems and potential solutions. *Health Psychology, 17,* 48-52.

Lobb, M. L., Shannon, M. C., Rrecer, S. L., & Allen, J. B. (1984). A behavioral technique for recovery from the psychological trauma of hysterectomy. *Perceptual & Motor Skills, 59,* 677-678.

Love, A. W. (1987). Depression in chronic low back pain patients: Diagnostic efficiency of three self-report questionnaires. *Journal of Clinical Psychology, 43,* 84 -89.

Lovibond, P. F., & Lovibond, S. H. (1995). The structure of negative emotional states: comparison of the Depression Anxiety Stress Scales (DASS) with the Beck Depression and Anxiety Inentories. *Behaviour Research and Therapy, 33,* 335-343.

Lowe, N. K. (1987). Individual variation in childbirth pain. *Journal of Psychosomatic Obstetrics & Gynecology, 7,* 183-192.

Lubin, B. (1965). Adjective check lists for measurement of depression. Archives of General Psychiatry, 12, 57-62.

Luborsky, L., & Auerbach, A. H. (1969). The symptom-context method. Quantitative studies of symptom formation in psychotherapy. *Journal of the American Psychoanalytic Association, 17,* 68-99.

Lumley, M. A., Torosian, T., Ketterer, M. W., & Pickard, S. D. (1997). Psychosocial factors related to noncardiac chest pain during treadmill exercise. *Psychosomatics, 38,* 230-238.

Lund, A. (1994). Neurochemical similarities in depression and pain, with special emphasis on serotonin. *Nordic Journal of Psychiatry, 48,* 419-428.

MacNeil, A. L., & Dick, W. C. (1976). Imipramine and rheumatoid factor. *Journal of International Medical Research, 4,* 23-27.

Maddock, R. J., Carter, C. S., Tavano-Hall, L., & Amsterdam, E. A. (1998). Hypocapnia associated with cardiac stress scintigraphy in chest pain patients with panic disorder. *Psychosomatic Medicine, 60,* 52-55.

Magni, G. (1984). Chronic low-back pain and depression: An epidemiological survey. *Acta Psychiatrica Scandinavica, 70*, 614-617.

Magni, G., Caldieron, C., Rigatti-Luchini, S., & Merskey, H. (1990). Chronic musculoskeletal pain and depressive symptoms in the general population: An analysis of the 1st National Health and Nutrition Examination Survey data. *Pain, 43*, 299-307.

Magni, G., Marchetti, M., Moreschi, C., & Merskey, H. (1993). Chronic musculoskeletal pain and depressive symptoms in the National Health and Nutrition Examination: I. Epidemiologic follow-up study. *Pain, 53*, 163-168.

Magni, G., Moreschi, C., Rigatti-Luchini, S., & Merskey, H. (1994). Prospective study on the relationship between depressive symptoms and chronic musculoskeletal pain. *Pain, 56*, 289-297.

Magni, G., Schifano, F., & de Leo, D. (1985). Pain as a symptom in elderly depressed patients: Relationship to diagnostic subgroups. *European Archives of Psychiatry & Neurological Sciences, 235*, 143-145.

Mairs, D. A. E. (1995). Hypnosis and pain in childbirth. *Contemporary Hypnosis, 12*, 111-118.

Malow, R. M. (1981). The effects of induced anxiety on pain perception: A signal detection analysis. *Pain, 11*, 397-405.

Malow, R. M., West, J. A., & Sutker, P. B. (1987). A sensory decision theory analysis of anxiety and pain responses in chronic drug abusers. *Journal of Abnormal Psychology, 96*, 184-189.

Malow, R. M., West, J. A., & Sutker, P. B. (1989). Anxiety and pain response changes across treatment: Sensory decision analysis. *Pain, 38*, 35-44

Mandke, R., Mishra, H., Kumaraiah, V., & Yavagal, S. T. (1996). Behavioural intervention in post-operative coronary heart disease patients. *NIMHANS Journal, 14*, 45-50.

Marbach, J. J., & Lund, P. (1981). Depression: Anhedonia and anxiety in temporomandibular joint and other facial pain syndromes. *Pain*, *11*, 73-84.

Marcussen, R. M., & Wolff, H. G. (1949). A formulation of the dynamics of the migraine headache. *Psychosomatic Medicine*, *11*, 251-256.

Marks, I. M. (1971). Phobic disorders four years after treatment: a prospective follow-up. *British Journal of Psychiatry*, *118*, 683-686.

Marsella, A. J., Hirschfeld, R. M. A., & Katz, M. M. (Eds.). *The measurement of depression* (pp. 87- 108). New York: Guilford.

Martelli, M. F., Auerbach, S. M., Alexander, J., & Mercuri, L. G. (1987). Stress management in the health care setting: Matching interventions with patient coping styles. *Journal of Consulting & Clinical Psychology*, *55*, 201-207.

Martin, P. R., & Teoh, H. J. (1999). Effects of visual stimuli and a stressor on head pain. *Headache*, *39*, 705-715.

Martinez-Urrutia, A. (1975). Anxiety and pain in surgical patients. *Journal of Consulting & Clinical Psychology*, *43*, 437-442.

Maruta, T., Swanson, D. W., & Swanson, W. M. (1976). Pain as a psychiatric symptom: Comparison between low back pain and depression. *Psychosomatics*, *17*, 123-127.

Maruta, T., Vatterott, M. K., & McHardy, M. J. (1989). Pain management as an antidepressant: Long-term resolution of pain-associated depression. *Pain*, *36*, 335-337.

Massie, M. J., & Holland, J. C. (1990). Depression and the cancer patient. *Journal of Clinical Psychiatry*, *51*, 12-19.

Max, M. (1994). Antidepressants as analgesics. In H. L. Fields & J. C. Liebeskind (Eds.), *Progress in pain research and management*, *vol.1. Pharmacological approaches to the treatment of chronic pain: New concepts and clinical issues* (pp. 229-246). Seattle: IASP Press.

Maxmen, J. S. (1991). *Psychotropic drugs: Fast facts*. New York: W. W. Norton.

Mayer, D. Y. (1975). Psychotropic drugs and the 'anti-depressed' personality. *British Journal of Medical Psychology*, *48*, 349 - 357.

Mayer, T. G., Gatchel, R. J., Kishino, N., Keeley, J., Capra, P., Mayer, H., Barnett, J., & Mooney, V. (1985). Objective assessment of spine function following industrial injury: A prospective study with comparison group and one-year follow-up. *Spine*, *10*, 482 - 493.

Mayeux, R., Stern, Y., Cote, L., & Williams, J. B. W. (1984). Altered seratonin metabolism in depressed patients with Parkinson's disease. *Neurology*, *34*, 642-646.

Mayou, R., & Hawton, K. (1986). Psychiatric disorder in the general hospital. *British Journal of Psychiatry*, *149*, 172-190.

McCracken, L.M. (1998). Learning to live with pain: Acceptance of pain predicts adjustment in persons with chronic pain. *Pain*, *74*, 21-27.

McCracken, L.M., & Gross, R.T. (1998). The role of pain-related anxiety reduction in the outcome of multidisciplinary treatment for chronic low back pain: Preliminary results. *Journal of Occupational Rehabilitation*, *8*, 179-189.

McCracken, L. M., Gross, R. T., Aikens, J, & Carnrike, C. L. M., Jr. (1996). The assessment of anxiety and fear in persons with chronic pain: A comparison of instruments. *Behaviour Research & Therapy*, *34*, 927-933.

McCracken, L. M., Gross, R. T., Sorg, P. J., Edmands, T. A., et al (1993). Prediction of pain in patients with chronic low back pain: Effects of inaccurate prediction and pain-related anxiety. *Behaviour Research & Therapy*, *31*, 647-652.

McCracken, L. M., Zayfert, C., & Gross, R. T. (1992). The Pain Anxiety Symptoms Scale: Development and validation of a scale to measure fear of pain. *Pain*, *50*, 67-73.

McCreary, C., Turner, J., & Dawson, E. (1977). Differences between functional versus organic low back pain patients. *Pain*, *4*, 73-78.

McDaniel, L. K., Anderson, K. O., Bradley, L. A., Turner, R. A., Agudelo, C. A., & Keefe, F. J. (1986). Development of an observational method for assessing pain behavior in rheumatoid arthritis. *Pain, 24*, 165-184.

McDonald Scott, W. A. (1969). The relief of pain with an anti-depressant in arthritis. *The Practitioner, 202*, 802 – 807.

McFarland, B. H., Freeborn, B. K., & Mullooly, J. P. (1985). Utilization patterns among long-term enrollees in a prepaid group practice health maintenance organization. *Medical Care, 23*, 1221-1233.

McKinley, J. C., & Hathaway, S. R. (1943). The identification and measurement of the psychoneuroses in medical practice: The Minnesota Multiphasic Personality Inventory. *Journal of the American Medical Association, 122*, 161-167.

McNair, D. M., Lorr, M., & Droppleman, L. F. (1981). *Profile of Mood States*. San Diego, CA: Educational and Industrial Testing Service.

McNeil, A. L., & Dick, W. L. (1976). Imipramine and rheumatoid factor. *Journal Int Med Res, 4*, 23 – 27.

McNeil, D. W., & Rainwater, A. J., III (1998). Development of the Fear of Pain Questionnaire--III. *Journal of Behavioral Medicine, 21*, 389-410

Meana, M. (1998). The meeting of pain and depression: Comorbidity in women. *Canadian Journal of Psychiatry, 43*, 893-899.

Meana, M., Binik, I., Khalife, S., & Cohen, D. (1998). Affect and marital adjustment in women's rating of dyspareunic pain. *Canadian Journal of Psychiatry, 43*, 381-385.

Meenan, R. F., Gertman, P. M., & Mason, J. R. (1980). Measuring health status in arthritis: The Arthritis Impact Measurement Scales: Further investigation of a health status measure. *Arthritis and Rheumatism, 25*, 1048-1053.

Megargee, E. I., Cook, P. E., & Mendelsohn, G. A. (1967). Development and validation of an MMPI scale of assaultiveness in overcontrolled individuals. *Journal of Abnormal Psychology, 72,* 519-528.

Meichenbaum, D., & Turk, D. C. (1976). The cognitive-behavioral management of anxiety, anger, and pain. In P.O. Davidson (Ed.), The behavioral management of anxiety, depression, and pain. New York: Brunner/Mazel.

Meilman, P. W. (1984). Chronic pain: The nature of the problem. *Journal of Orthopaedic & Sports Physical Therapy, 5,* 307-308.

Melding, P. S. (1995). How do older people respond to chronic pain? A review of coping with pain and illness in elders. *Pain Reviews, 2,* 65-75.

Mellsop, G. W., Hutton, J. D., & Delahunt, J. W. (1985). Dexamethasone suppression test as a simple measure of stress? *British Medical Journal Clinical Resident Edition, 290,* 1804-1806.

Melzack, R. (1975). The McGill Pain Questionnaire: Major properties and scoring methods. *Pain, 1,* 277-299.

Melzack, R. & Casey, K. L. (1968). Sensory, motivational, and central control of determinants of pain. In D. R. Kenshalo (Ed.), *The skin senses* (pp. 423-439). Springfield, IL: Charles C. Thomas.

Mendel, C. M., Klein, R. F., & Chappell, D. A. (1986). A trial of amitripyline and fluphenazine in the treatment of painful diabetic neuropathy. *JAMA, 255,* 637-639.

Mendels, J., & Weinstein, N. (1972). The relationship between depression and anxiety. *Archives of General Psychiatry, 27,* 649-653.

Merskey, H. & Moulin, D. (1999). Pharmacological treatment in chronic pain. In A. R. Block, E. F. Kremer, & E. Fernandez (Eds.), *Handbook of pain syndromes.* New Jersey: Lawrence Erlbaum Associates, Inc.

Merskey, H. (1965). The characteristics of persistent pain in psychological illness. *Journal of Psychosomatic Research, 9,* 291-298.

Merskey, H. (1986). Classification of chronic pain: Descriptions of chronic pain syndromes and definitions. *Pain*, S1-S225.

Merskey, H. (1993). Chronic muscular pain: A life stress syndrome? *Journal of Musculoskeletal Pain*, *1*, 61-69.

Merskey, H., & Hester, R. A. (1972). The treatment of chronic pain with psychotropic drugs. *Postgraduate Medical Journal*, *48*, 594-598.

Millstein, S. G., Adler, N. E., & Irwin, C.E. (1984). Sources of anxiety about pelvic examinations among adolescent females. *Journal of Adolescent Health Care*, *5*, 105-111

Moffic, H. S., & Paykel, E. S. (1975). Depression in medical in-patients. *British Journal of Psychiatry*, *126*, 346-353.

Mohamed, S. N., Weisz, G. M., & Waring, E. M. (1978). The relationship of chronic pain to depression, marital adjustment, and family dynamics. *Pain*, *5*, 285-292.

Molchan, S. E., Lawlor, B. A., Hill, J. L., & Martinez, R. A. (1991). CSF monoamine metabolites and somatostatin in Alzheimer's disease and major depression. *Biological Psychiatry*, *29*, 1110-1118.

Moldofsky, H., & Chester, W. (1970). Pain and mood patterns in patients with rheumatoid arthritis: A prospective study. *Psychosomatic Medicine*, *32*, 309-318.

Montgomery, S. A., & Asberg, M. (1979). A new depression scale designed to be sensitive to change. *British Journal of Psychiatry, 134*, 382-389.

Monti, D. A., Herring, C. L., Schwartzman, R. J., & Marchese, M. (1998). Personality assessment of patients with Complex Regional Pain Syndrome Type I. *Clinical Journal of Pain*, *14*, 295-302.

Moore, D. P. (1980). Treatment of chronic pain with tricyclic anti-depressants. *Southern Medical Journal*, *73*, 1585 – 1586.

Morgan, W. P., & Horstman, D. H. (1978). Psychometric correlates of pain perception. *Perceptual & Motor Skills*, *47*, 27-39.

Morillo, E., & Gardner, L. I. (1979). Bereavement as an antecedent factor in thyrotoxicosis of childhood: Four case studies with survey of possible metabolic pathways. *Psychosomatic Medicine, 41*, 545-555.

Moss, M. S., Lawton, M. P., & Gliscksman, A. (1991). The role of pain in the last year of life of older persons. *Journal of Gerontology: Psychological Sciences, 46*, 51 - 57.

Munafo', M. R. (1978). Perioperative anxiety and postoperative pain. *Psychology, Health & Medicine, 3*, 429-433

Muris, P., de Jongh, A., van Zuuren, F. J., Ter Horst, G, et al (1995). Imposed and chosen monitoring and blunting strategies in the dental setting: Effects, self-efficacy, and coping preference. *Anxiety, Stress & Coping: An International Journal, 8*, 47-59.

Murphy, E., Smith, R., Lindesay, J., & Slattery, J. (1988). *British Journal of Psychiatry, 152*, 347-353.

Naidoo, P., & Pillay, Y. G. (1994). Correlations among general stress, family environment, psychological distress, and pain experience. *Perceptual & Motor Skills, 78*, 1291-1296.

Nelson, F. V., Zimmerman, L., Barnason, S., Nieveen, J., & Schmaderer, M. (1998). The relationship and influence of anxiety on postoperative pain in the coronary artery bypass graft patient. *Journal of Pain & Symptom Management, 15*, 102-109.

Nelson, W. M. (1981). A cognitive-behavioral treatment for disproportionate dental anxiety and pain: A case study. *Journal of Clinical Child Psychology, 10*, 79-82.

Nezu, A.M., McClure, K.S., Ronan, G., & Meadows, E.A. (Eds.) (2000). Practitioner's guide to empirically-based measures of depression. Norwell, MA: Kluwer.

Nicassio, P. M, Schuman, C., Radojevic, V., & Weisman, M. H. (1999). Helplessness as a mediator of health status in fibromyalgia. *Cognitive Therapy and Research, 23*, 181 - 196.

Nicassio, P. M., & Wallston, K. A. (1992). Longitudinal relationships among pain , sleep, and depression in rheumatoid arthritis. *Journal of Abnormal Psychology, 101*, 514-520.

Nilsson, H. L., & von Knorring, L. (1989). Review: Clomipramine in acute and chronic pain syndromes. *Nordisk Psykiatrisk Tidsskrift, (Suppl. 20),* 101-113.

Nolan, T. E., Metheny, W. P., & Smith, R. P. (1992). Unrecognized association of sleep disorders and depression with chronic pelvic pain. *Southern Medical Journal, 85,* 1181-1183.

Noone, J. F. (1977). Psychotropic drugs and migraine. Journal of Internal Medicine Research, 5, 66 – 71.

Novaco, R. W. (1974). *The effect of disposition for anger and degree of provocation on self-report and physiological measures of anger in various modes of provocation.* Unpublished manuscript, Indiana University, Bloomington, IN.

Novy, D. M., Nelson, D. V., Berry, L. A., & Averill, P. M. (1995). What does the Beck Depression Inventory measure in chronic pain? A reappraisal. *Pain, 61,* 261-267.

Oberle, K., Paul, P., Wry, J., & Grace, M. (1992). Pain, anxiety, and analgesics: A comparative study of elderly and younger surgical patients. *Canadian Journal on Aging, 9,* 13-22.

Oest, L-G. (1987). Applied relaxation: Description of a coping technique and review of controlled studies. *Behaviour Research & Therapy, 25,* 397-409.

Okifuji, A., Turk, D. C., & Curran, S. L. (1999). Anger in chronic pain: Investigations of anger targets and intensity. *Journal of Psychosomatic Research, 47,* 1-12.

Onghena, P., & Van Houdenhove, B. (1992). Antidepressant-induced analgesia in chronic non-malignant pain: a meta-analysis of 39 placebo-controlled studies. *Pain, 49,* 205-220.

Onghena, P., de Cuyper, H.; Van Houdenhove, B.; Verstraeten, D. (1993). Mianserin and chronic pain: A double-blind placebo-controlled process and outcome study. *Acta Psychiatrica Scandinavica, 88,* 198-204.

Ortony, A., Clore, G., & Collins, A. (1988). *The cognitive structure of emotions*. Cambridge, England: Cambridge University Press.

Osman, A., Barrios, F.X., Osman, J.R., Schneekloth, R, et al. (1994). The Pain Anxiety Symptoms Scale: Psychometric properties in a community sample. *Journal of Behavioral Medicine, 17*, 511-522

Owen-Salters, E., Gatchel, R. J., Polatin, P. B., & Mayer, T. G. (1996). Changes in psychopathology following functional restoration of chronic low back pain patients: A prospective study. *Journal of Occupational Rehabilitation, 6*, 215-223.

Paanksep (1994). The basics of basic emotion. In P. Ekman & R.J. Davidson (Eds.), *The nature of emotion: Fundamental questions* (pp. 20-24). New York: Oxford University Press.

Palermo, T. M., & Drotar, D. (1996). Prediction of children's post-operative pain: The role of presurgical expectations and anticipatory emotions. *Journal of Pediatric Psychology, 21*, 683-698.

Pancheri, P., Zichella, L., Fraioli, F., Carilli, L., Perrone, G., Biondi, M., Fabbri, A., Santoro, A., & Moretti, C. (1985). ACTH, beta-endorphin and met-enkephalin: Peripheral modifications during the stress of human labor. *Psycho-neuroendocrinology, 10*, 289-301.

Paoli, F., Darcourt, G., & Corsa, P. (1960). Note preliminaire sure l'action de l'imipramine don les etats douloureaux. *Revue Neurologique, 102*, 503 – 504.

Parmelee, P. A., Katz, I. R., & Lawton, M. P. (1991). The relation of pain to depression among institutionalized aged. *Journals of Gerontology, 46*, P15-P21

Paul, G. L. (1966). Insight versus. Desensitization in psychotherapy. Stanford, CA: Stanford University Press.

Peck, J. R., Smith, T. W., Ward, J. R., & Milano, F. (1989). Disability and depression in rheumatoid arthritis: A multitrait-multimethod investigation. *Arthritis and Rheumatism, 32*, 1100-1106.

Pelz, M., Merskey, H., Brant, C. C., & Heseltine, GFD. (1981). A note on the occurrence of pain in psychiatric patients from a Canadian Indian and Inuit population. *Pain, 10,* 75-78.

Pennebaker, J. W. (1989). Confession, inhibition, and disease. In L. Berkowitz (Ed.), *Advances in experimental social psychology* (Vol. 22), (pp. 211-244). Orlando, FL: Academic Press.

Pennebaker, J. W. (1992). Inhibition as the linchpin of health. In H. S. Friedman (Ed.), *Hostility, coping and health* (pp. 127-139). Washington D.C.: American Psychological Association.

Perl, E. R. (1980). Afferent basis of nociception and pain: evidence from the characteristics of sensory receptors and their projections to the spinal dorsal horn. In J. J. Bonica (Ed), *Pain.* New York: Raven Press.

Philips, H. C. (1989). Thoughts provoked by pain. *Behaviour Research and Therapy, 27,* 469-473.

Philips, H. C., & Jahanshahi, M. (1985). The effects of persistent pain: The chronic headache sufferer. *Pain, 21,* 163 - 176.

Philips, H. C., & Grant, L. (1991). The evolution of chronic back pain problems: A longitudinal study. *Behaviour Research & Therapy, 29,* 435-441.

Philips, H. C., & Rachman, S. (1996). The psychological management of chronic pain: A treatment manual. New York: Springer Publishing Company.

Pickett, C., & Clum, G. A. (1982). Comparative treatment strategies and their interaction with locus of control in the reduction of postsurgical pain and anxiety. *Journal of Consulting & Clinical Psychology, 50,* 439-441.

Piercy, M., Elithorn, A., Pratt, R. T. C., & Crosskey, M. (1982). Anxiety and an autonomic reaction to pain. *Journal of Neurology, Neurosurgery & Psychiatry, 18,* 155-162.

Pilling, L. F., Brannick, T. L., & Swenson, W. M. (1967). Psychologic characteristics of psychiatric patients having pain as a presenting symptom. *Canadian Medical Association Journal, 97*, 387-394.

Pilowsky (1988). Affective disorders and pain. In R. Dubner, G. F. Gebhart & M. R. Bond (Eds.), *Proceedings of the Vth World Congress on Pain* (pp.263-275). Amsterdam: Elsevier.

Pilowsky, I. (1989). Pain and illness behavior: Assessment and management. In P. D. Wall and R. Melzack (Eds.), Textbook of pain (2nd edition), pp. 980-988). Edinburgh: Churchill Livingstone.

Pilowsky, I., & Spence, N. (1976). Pain, anger and illness behaviour. *Journal of Psychosomatic Research, 20*, 411-416.

Pilowsky, I., & Spence, N. D. (1983). Manual for the Illness Behaviour Questionnaire (IBQ) (2nd ed.). Adelaide, South Australia: University of Adelaide.

Pilowsky, I., Crettenden, I., & Townley, M. (1985). Sleep disturbance in pain clinic patients. *Pain, 23*, 27-33.

Pincus, T., & Williams, A. (1999). Models and measurements of depression in chronic pain. *Journal of Psychosomatic Research, 47*, 211-219.

Pincus, T., Callahan, L. F., Bradley, L. A., Vaugh W. K., & Wolfe, F. (1986). Elevated MMPI scores for hypocondrasis, depression, and hysteria in patients with rheumatoid arthritis reflect disease rather than psychological status. *Arthritis and Rheumatism, 29*, 1456-1466.

Pincus, T., Fraser, L., & Pearce, S. Do chronic pain patients "Stroop" on pain stimuli? *British Journal of Clinical Psychology, 37*, 49-58.

Pincus, T., Pearce, S., & McClelland, A. (1995). Endorsement and memory bias of self-referential pain stimuli in depressed pain patients. *British Journal of Clinical Psychology, 34*, 267-277.

Price, D. D. (1999). *Psychological mechanisms of pain and analgesia*. Seattle, Washington: IASP Press.

Price, D. D., & Harkins, S. W. (1992). The affective-motivational dimension of pain. *American Pain Society Journal, 1*, 229-239.

Rabkin, J. G., & Klein, D. F. (1987). The clinical measurement of depressive disorders. In A. J. Marsella, R. M. A. Hirschfeld, & M. M. Katz (Eds.), The measurement of depression (pp. 30-83). New York: Guilford Press.

Radloff, L. S. (1977) The CES-D scale: a self-report depression scale for research in the general population. *Applied Psychological Measurement, 1*, 385-401.

Radloff, L. S., & Teri, L. (1986). Use of the Center for Epidemiological Studies-Depression scale with older adults. In *Clinical gerontology* (pp. 119-136). New Jersey: Rutgers University Press.

Randall, G., Ewalt, J., & Blair, H. (1945). Psychiatric reaction to amputation. *Journal of the American Medical Association, 128*, 645.

Rapee, R. M. (1991). Generalized anxiety disorder: A review of clinical features and theoretical concepts. *Clinical Psychology Review, 11*, 419-440.

Rapee, R. M. (1993). Psychological factors in panic disorder. *Advances in Behaviour Research and Therapy, 15*, 85-102.

Raphael, K. G., & Marbach, J. J. (1997). When did your pain start?: Reliability of self-reported age of onset of facial pain. *Clinical Journal of Pain, 13,* 352-359.

Rasmussen, P. R., & Jeffrey, A. C. (1995). Assessment of mood states: Biases in single-administration assessments. *Journal of Psychopathology and Behavioral Assessment, 17*, 177-184.

Reading, A. E., & Cox, D. N. (1985). Psychosocial predictors of labor pain. *Pain, 22*, 309-315.

Reesor, K. A., & Craig, K. D. (1988). Medically incongruent chronic back pain: Physical limitations, suffering, and ineffective coping. *Pain, 32*, 35-45.

Regier, D. A., Boyd, J. H., Burke, J. D., & Rae, D. S. (1988). One-month prevalence of mental Relation to depression and disability. *Journal of Consulting & Clinical Psychology, 56,* 412-416.

Relationship between social desirability and self-report in chronic pain patients. *Clinical Journal of Pain, 11,* 189-193.

Reynolds, W. M., & Kobak, K. A. (1995). *Hamilton Depression Inventory.* Odesa, FL: Psychological Assessment Resources.

Reynolds, W. M., & Kobak, K. A. (1995). Hamilton Depression Inventory. Odesa, FL: Psychological Assessment Resources.

Richeimer, M. D., Bajwa, Z. H., Kahraman, S. S., Ransil, B. J., & Warfield, C. W. (1997). Utilization patterns of tricyclic antidepressants in a multidisciplinary pain clinic: A survey. *The Clinical Journal of Pain, 13,* 324 - 329.

Rizzo, P.A, et al. (1985). Pain, anxiety, and contingent negative variation: A clinical and pharmacological study. *Biological Psychiatry, 20,* 1297-1302.

Robinson, R. G., & Price, T. R. (1982). Post-stroke depressive disorders: A follow-up study of 103 patients. *Stroke, 13,* 653-641.

Robinson, R. G., Starr, L. B., Kubos, K. L., & Prince, T. R. (1983). A two-year longitudinal study of post-stroke mood disorders: Findings during the initial evaluation. *Stroke, 14,* 736-741.

Rodgers, L. (1995). Music for surgery. *Advances, 11,* 49-57.

Rodin, G., & Voshart, K. (1987). Depressive symptoms and functional impairment in the medically ill. *General Hospital Psychiatry, 9,* 251-258.

Rodin, G., Craven, J., & Littlefield, C. (1991). Depression in the medically ill: An integrated approach. New York: Brunner Mazel.

Rollman, G. B. (1991). Pain responsiveness. In M. A. Heller & W. Schiff (Eds.), *The psychology of touch.* Hillsdale, NJ: Lawrence Erlbaum & Associates.

Rollman, G. B. (1998). Culture and pain. In S. Kazarian & D. R. Evans (Eds.), *Cultural clinical psychology: Theory, research, and practice* (pp. 267-286). New York: Oxford University Press.

Romano, J. M., & Turner, J. A. (1985). Chronic pain and depression: Does the evidence support a relationship? *Psychological Bulletin, 97*, 18-34.

Roose, S. P., Glassman, A. H., Siris, S., Walsh, B. T., Bruno, R. L., & Wright, L.B. (1981). Comparison of imipramine and nortriptyline-induced orthostatic hypotension: a meaningful difference. *Journal of Clinical Pharmacology, 1*, 316-319.

Roseman, I. J. (1991). Appraisal determinants of discrete emotions. *Cognition and Emotion, 5*, 161-200.

Rosenbaum, J. F. (1982). Comments on "chronic pain as a variant of depressive disease: The pain-prone disorder." *Journal of Nervous and Mental Diseases, 170*, 412-414.

Rosenberg, S. J., Peterson, R. A., Hayes, J. R., Hatcher, J., & Headen, S. (1988). Depression in medical in-patients. *British Journal of Medical Psychology, 61*, 245-254.

Rosenzweig, S. (1976). Aggressive behavior and the Rosenzweig picture frustration study. *Journal of Clinical Psychology, 32*, 885-891.

Rosenzweig, S. (1978). *The Rosenzweig Picture-Frustration (P-F) Study basic manual and adult form supplement*. St. Louis: Rana.

Ross, D. M. (1985). Thought-stopping: A coping strategy for impending feared events. *Issues in Comprehensive Pediatric Nursing, 7*, 83-89.

Ross, M. J., & Berger, R. (1996). Scott Effects of stress inoculation training on athletes' postsurgical pain and rehabilitation after orthopedic injury. *Journal of Consulting & Clinical Psychology, 64*, 406-410.

Rotter, J. (1966). Generalized expectancies for internal versus external control of reinforcement. *Psychological Monographs, 80*, 609.

Roy, R. (1982-1983). Many faces of depression in patients with chronic pain. *International Journal of Psychiatry in Medicine, 12,* 109-119.

Roy, R. (1986-1987). Measurement of chronic pain in pain-depression literature during the 1980s: A review. *International Journal of Psychiatry in Medicine, 16,* 179-188.

Roy, R., Thomas, M., & Matas, M. (1984). Chronic pain and depression: A review. *Comprehensive Psychiatry, 25,* 96-105.

Roy-Byrne, P., Uhde, T. W., Post, R. M., King, A. C., & Buchsbaum, M. S. (1985). Normal pain sensitivity in patients with panic disorder. *Psychiatry Research, 14,* 77-84.

Rudy, T. E., Kerns, R. D., & Turk, D. C. (1988). Chronic pain and depression: Toward a cognitive-behavioral mediation model. *Pain, 35,* 129-140.

Rugh, J. D., Hatch, J. P., Moore, P. J., Cyr-Provost, M., Boutros, N. N., & Pellegrino, C. S. (1990). The effects of psycho-social stress on electromyographic activity and negative affect in ambulatory tensio-type headache patients. *Headache, 30,* 216-219.

Sacher, J. B. (1983). Coping and living with herpes. *Journal of the American College of Health, 31,* 261-262.

Sagduyu, A. & Sahiner, T. (1997). Psychiatric disorders in patients with migraine and tension-type headache. *Tuerk Psikiyatri Dergisi, 8,* 45-49.

Salter, J. R. (1985). Gynaecological symptoms and psychological distress in potential hysterectomy patients. *Source Journal of Psychosomatic Research, 29,* 155-159.

Sandford, J. J., Argyropoulos, S. V., & Nutt, D. J. (2000). The psychobiology of anxiolytic drugs. Part 1: Basic neurobiology. *Pharmacology and therapeutics, 88,* 197-212.

Schacham, S. A. (1983). A shortened version of the Profile of Mood States. *Journal of Personality Assessment, 47,* 305-307.

Schafer, M. (1994). Typus melancholicus as a personality characteristic of migraine patients. *European Archives of Psychiatry and Clinical Neuroscience, 243*, 328 - 339.

Schaffer, C. B., Donlon, P. T., & Bittle, R. M. (1980). Chronic pain and depression: A clinical and family history survey. *American Journal of Psychiatry, 137*, 118-120.

Schalling, D., & Levander, S. (1964). Ratings of anxiety-proneness and responses to electrical pain stimulation. *Scandinavian Journal of Psychology, 5*, 1-9.

Scherer (1994). Toward a concept of "modal emotions". In P. Ekman & R. J. Davidson (Ed.), *The nature of emotion: Fundamental questions* (pp. 25-31). New York: Oxford University Press.

Scherwitz, L., & Rugulies, R. (1992). Life-style and hostility. In H. S. Friedman (Ed.), *Hostility, coping, and health* (pp. 77-98). Washington, DC: American Psychological Association.

Schisler, T., Lander, J., & Fowler-Kerry, S. (1998). *Journal of Pain & Symptom Management, 16*, 80-87

Schmale, A. H., & Iker, H. (1971). Hopelessness as a predictor of cervical cancer. *Social Science & Medicine, 5*, 95-100.

Schmale, A. H. (1972). Depression as affect, character style, and symptom formation. *Psychoanalysis & Contemporary Science, 1*, 327-351 .

Schmidt, J. P., & Wallace, R. W. (1982). Factorial analysis of the MMPI profiles of low back pain patients. *Journal of Personality Assessment, 46*, 366-369.

Schocken, D. D., Greene, A. F., Worden, T. J., Harrison, E. E., et al. (1987). Effects of age and gender on the relationship between anxiety and coronary artery disease. *Psycho-somatic Medicine, 49*, 118-126

Schonfeld, L. (1982). Covert assertion as a method for coping with pain and pain related behaviors. *Clinical Gerontologist, 12*, 17-29.

Schonfeld, W. H., Verboncoeur, C. J., Fifer, S. K., Lipschutz, R. C., Lubeck, D. P., & Buesching, D. P. (1997). The functioning and well-being of patients with unrecognized anxiety disorders and major depressive disorder. *Journal of Affective Disorders, 43*, 105 - 119.

Schulberg, H.C., Saul, M., McClelland, M., Ganguli, M., Christy, W., & Frank, R. (1985). Assessing depression in primary medical and psychiatric practices. *Archives of General Psychiatry, 42*, 1164-1170.

Schultz, J. H. (1932). Das autogene training-konzentrative selbstentspannung. Versuch einer Klinisch-praktischen darstellung. Stuttgart: Thieme.

Schumacher, R., & Velden, M. (1984). Anxiety, pain experience, and pain report: A signal-detection study. *Perceptual & Motor Skills, 58*, 339-349.

Schwab, J. J., Bialow, M. R., & Clemmons, R. S., & Holzer, C. E. (1967). The affective symptomatology of depression in medical inpatients. *Psychosomatic Medicine, 7*, 214-217.

Schwartz, L., Slater, M., Birchler, G., & Atkinson, J. (1991). Depression in spouses of chronic pain patients: The role of pain and anger, and marital satisfaction. *Pain, 44*, 61-67.

Schwartz-Barcott, D., Fortin, J. D., & Kim, H. S.. (1994). Clienturse interaction: Testing for its impact in preoperative instruction. *International Journal of Nursing Studies, 31*, 23-35.

Seligman, M. E. P. (1975). *Helplessness: On depression, development, and death.* San Francisco: Freeman.

Serlie, A. W., Duivenvoorden, H. J., Passchier, J., ten Cate, F. J., et al (1996). Empirical psychological modeling of chest pain: A comparative study. *Journal of Psychosomatic Research, 40*, 625-635.

Shacham, S., & Daut, R. (1981). Anxiety or pain: What does the scale measure? *Journal of Consulting & Clinical Psychology, 49*, 468-469.

Sherman, R. A., Sherman, C. J., & Bruno, G. M. (1987) Psychological factors influencing chronic phantom limb pain: An analysis of the literature. *Pain, 28,* 285-295.

Sherman, R. A., Gall, N., & Gormly, J. (1979). Treatment of phantom limb pain with muscular relaxation training to disrupt the pain^anxiety^tension cycle. *Pain, 6,* 47-55.

Shiloh, S., Mahlev, U., Dar, R., & Ben-Rafael, Z. (1998). Interactive effects of viewing a contraction monitor and information-seeking style on reported childbirth pain. *Cognitive Therapy & Research, 22,* 501-516.

Shiomi, K. (1978). Relations of pain threshold and pain tolerance in cold water with scores on Maudsley Personality Inventory and Manifest Anxiety Scale. *Perceptual & Motor Skills, 47,* 1155-1158.

Shukla, G., Sahu, S., Tripathi, R., & Gupta, D. (1982). A psychiatric study of amputees. *British Journal of Psychiatry, 141,* 50-53.

Siegel, J. M. (1986). The Multidimensional Anger Inventory. *Journal of Personality and Social Psychology, 51,* 191-200.

Siegel, K., Kalb, R., & Pasternak, G. W. (1983). Analgesic activity of tricyclic antidepressants. *Ann. Neurology, 13,* 462-465.

Sifneos, P. E. (1973). The prevalence of alexithymic characteristics in psychosomatic patients. *Psychotherapy and Psychosomatics, 22,* 255 - 262.

Silber, E.; Rey, A. C.; Savard, R. & Post, R. M. (1980). Thought disorder and affective inaccessibility in depression. *Journal of Clinical Psychiatry, 41,* 161-165.

Singh, G. (1968). The diagnosis of depression. *Punjab Medical Journal, 18,* 53-59.

Sinyor, D., Amato, P., Kaloupek, D.G., Becker, R., Goldenberg, M., & Coopersmith, H. (1986). Post-stroke depression: Relationships to functional impairment, coping strategies, and rehabilitation outcome. *Stroke, 17,* 1102-1107.

Skevington, S. M. (1993). Depression and causal attributions in the early stages of a chronic painful disease: A longitudinal study of early synovitis. *Psychology & Health*, *8*, 51-64.

Skiffington, S., Fernandez, E., & McFarland, K. A. (1998). Towards the validation of multiple features in the assessment of emotions. *European Journal of Psychological Assessment*, *14*, 202-210.

Skinner, B. F. (1953). *Science and human behavior of organisms.* New York: Macmillan.

Slocumb, J. C., Kellner, R., Rosenfeld, R. C., & Pathak, D. Anxiety and depression in patients with the abdominal pelvic pain syndrome. *General Hospital Psychiatry*, *11*, 48-53.

Smedslund, J. (1992). How shall the concept of anger be defined? *Theory and Psychology*, *3*, 5-34.

Smith, G. R. (1992). The epidemiology and treatment of depression when it coexists with somatoform disorders, somatization, or pain. *General Hospital Psychiatry*, *14*, 265-272.

Smith, G. C., Clarke, D. M., Handrinos, D., & Dunsis, D. (1998). Consultation-liaison psychiatrists' management of depression. *Psychosomatics*, *39*, 244 - 252.

Smith, J. T., Barabasz, A., & Barabasz, M. (1996). Comparison of hypnosis and distraction in severely ill children undergoing painful medical procedures. *Journal of Counseling Psychology*, *43*, 187-195.

Smith, T. W., & Christensen, A. J. (1992). Hostility, health, and social contexts. In H. S. Friedman (Ed.), *Hostility, coping, and health* (pp.33-48). Washington, DC: American Psychological Association.

Smith, T. W., Christensen, A. J., Peck, J. R., & Ward, J. R. (1994). Cognitive distortion, helplessness, and depressed mood in rheumatoid arthritis: A four-year longitudinal analysis. *Health Psychology*, *13*, 213-217

Smith, T. W., Peck, J. R., Milano, R. A., & Ward, J. R. (1988). Cognitive distortion in rheumatoid arthritis: Disorders in the United States: Based on five epidemiologic catchment area sites. *Archives of General Psychiatry, 45,* 977-986.

Smith, T. W., Pope, M. K., Sanders, J. D., Allred, K. D., & O'Keefe, J. L. (1988). Cynical hostility at home and work: Psychosocial vulnerability across domains. *Journal of Research in Personality, 25,* 525-548.

Smits, D. J., De Boeck, P., Kuppens, P., & Van Mechelen, I. (2002). The structure of negative emotion scales: Generalization over contexts and comprehensiveness. *European Journal of Personality, 16,* 127-141.

Snaith, R. P., Ahmed, S. N., Melita, M. C., & Hamilton, M. (1971). The investment of severity of primary depressive illness. *Psychological Medicine, 1,* 153-159.

Snekelle, R., Raynor, W., Ostfeld, A., Garron, D., Bieliauskas, L., Shuguey, L., Muliza, C., & Oglesby, P. (1981). Psychological depression and 17 year risk of death from cancer. *Psychosomatic Medicine, 43,* 117-125.

Sokel, B., Lansdown, R., Kent, A. (1990). The development of a hypnotherapy service for children. *Child: Care, Health & Development, 16,* 227-233

Sorkin, B. A., Rudy, T. E., Hanlon, R. B., Turk, D. C., & Steig, R. L. (1990). Chronic pain in old and young patients: differences appear less important than similarities. *Journal of Gerontology, 45,* 64-68.

Spear, F. G. (1967). Pain in psychiatric patients. *Journal of Psychosomatic Research, 11,* 187-193.

Spence, J. E., Olson, M. (1997). Quantitative research on therapeutic touch: An integrative review of the literature 1985-1995. *Scandinavian Journal of Caring Sciences, 11,* 183-190.

Spence, S. H. (1989). Cognitive-behavior therapy in the management of chronic, occupational pain of the upper limbs. *Behaviour Research & Therapy, 27,* 435-446.

Spencer, P. S. J. (1976). Some aspects of the pharmacology of analgesia. *Journal of Internal. Med. Res, 4,* 1-14.

Spielberger, C. D. (1988). *State-Trait Anger Expression Inventory Professional Manual.* Odessa, FL: Psychological Assessment Resources, Inc.

Spielberger, C. D. (1999). The State-Trait Anger Expression Inventory-2 Professional Manual. Odessa, FL: Psychological Assessment Resources, Inc.

Spielberger, C. D., & Sydeman, S.J. (1993). State-trait anxiety inventory and state-trait anger expression inventory. In M. E. Maruish (Ed.), *The use of psychological tests for treatment planning and outcome assessment* (pp. 292-321). Hillsdale, NJ: Lawrence Erlbaum.

Spielberger, C. D., Gorsuch, S. L., & Lushene, R. E. (1970). Manual for the State-Trait Anxiety Inventory (self-evaluation questionnaire). Palo Alto, CA: Consulting Psychologists Press.

Spielberger C. D., Gorsuch, R. L., Lushene, R. E., Vagg, P. R., & Jacobs, G. A. (1977). The state-trait anxiety inventory: Test manual for form Y. Palo Alto, CA: Consulting Psychologists Press.

Spielberger, C. D., Jacobs, G., Crane, R., Russell, S., Westberry, L., Barker, L., Johnson, E., Knight, J., & Marks, E. (1979). *Preliminary manual for the State-Trait Personality Inventory (STPI).* Tampa: University of South Florida Human Resources Institute.

Spielberger, C. D., Jacobs, G., Russell, S., & Crane, R. S. (1983). Assessment of anger: The state-trait anger scale. In J. N. Butcher & C. D. Spielberger (Eds.), *Advances in personality assessment. (Vol. 2)* (pp. 159-186). Hillsdale, NJ: Lawrence Erlbaum.

Spielberger, C. D., Johnson, E. H., Russell, S. F., Crane, R. J., Jacobs, G. A., & Worden, T. J. (1985). The experience and expression of anger: Construction and validation of an anger expression scale.   In M. A. Chesney & R. H. Rosenman (Eds.), *Anger and hostility in cardiovascular and behavioral disorders* (pp. 5-30). New York: Hemisphere/McGraw-Hill.

Spielberger, C. D., Krasner, S. S., & Solomon, E. P. (1988). The experience, expression and control of anger. In M.P. Janisse (Ed.), *Health Psychology: Individual differences and stress.* (pp. 89-108). New York: Springer-Verlag.

Spitzer, R. L., Endicott, J., & Robins, E. (1978). Research Diagnostic Criteria: rationale and reliability. *Archives of General Psychiatry, 35,* 773-782.

Spitzer, R. L., Williams, J. B.W., Gibbon, M., & First, M. B. (1992). The Structured Clinical Interview for DSM-III-R (SCID): I. History, rationale, and description. *Archives of General Psychiatry, 49,* 624-629.

Stam, H. J., McGrath, P. A., Brooke, R. I. (1984). The treatment of temporomandibular joint syndrome through control of anxiety. *Journal of Behavior Therapy & Experimental Psychiatry, 15,* 41-45.

Staufer, J. D. (1987). Antidepressants and chronic pain. *Journal of Family Practice, 25,* 167-170.

Stein, D. J., & Young, J. E. (1992). *Cognitive science and clinical disorders.* San Diego: Academic Press.

Sternbach, R. (1968). *Pain: A psychophysiological analysis.* Academic Press, New York.

Sternbach, R. A. (1975). Psychophysiology of pain. *International Journal of Psychiatry in Medicine, 6,* 63-73.

Sternbach, R. A., Wolf, S. R., Murphy, R. W., & Akeson, W. H. (1973). Aspects of chronic low back pain. *Psychosomatics, 14,* 52-56.

Sternbach, R. A., Wolf, S. R., Murphy, R. W., & Akeson, W. H. (1973). Traits of pain patients: The low-back "losers". *Psychosomatics, 14,* 226-229.

Stone, A. A., & Neale, J. M. (1984). Effects of severe daily events on mood. *Journal of Personality & Social Psychology, 46,* 137-144.

Stone, A. A., & Shiffman, S. (1994). Ecological momentary assessment (EMA) in behavorial medicine. *Annals of Behavioral Medicine, 16,* 199-202.

Stone, A. A., Jandorf, L., & Neale, J. M. (1986). Triggers or aggravators of symptoms? *Social Science & Medicine, 22,* 1015-1018.

Stone, A. A., Reed, B. R., & Neale, J. M. (1987). Changes in daily event frequency precede episodes of physical symptoms. *Journal of Human Stress, 13,* 70-74.

Stone, A. A.; Schwartz, J. E.; Neale, J. M.; Shiffman, S; Marco, C. A.; Hickcox, M., Paty, J., Porter, L. S., & Cruise, L. J. (1998). A comparison of coping assessed by ecological momentary assessment and retrospective recall. *Journal of Personality & Social Psychology, 74,* 1670-1680.

Strang, P. (1987). Existential consequences of unrelieved cancer pain. *Palliative Medicine, 11,* 299-305.

Suinn, R. (2001).   The terrible twos -- Anger and Anxiety. *American Psychologist, 56,* 27-36.

Sullivan, M. J., Reesor, K., Mikail, S., & Fisher, R. (1992). The treatment of depression in chronic low back pain: Review and recommendations. *Pain, 50,* 5-13.

Sullivan, M. J. L, & D'Eon, J. (1990). Relation between catastrophizing and depression in chronic pain patients. *Journal of Abnormal Psychology, 99,* 260 - 263.

Summers, J. D., Rapoff, M. A., Varghese, G., Porter, K., & Palmer, P. (1991). Psychosocial factors in chronic spinal cord injury pain. *Pain, 47,* 183-189.

Svobodova, J., & Trnka, J. (1997). Breathing in the treatment of anxiety neurosis and polyalgic syndrome. *Studia Psychologica, 39,* 328-329.

Swanson, David W.; Maruta, Toshihiko; Wolff, Virginia A. (1986). Ancient pain. *Pain, 25,* 383-387.

Taenzer, P., Melzack, R., & Jeans, M. E. (1986). Influence of psychological factors on postoperative pain, mood and analgesic requirements. *Pain, 24,* 331-342.

Tait, R. C., Chibnall, J. T., & Margolis, R. B. (1990). Pain extent: Relations with psychological state, pain severity, pain history, and disability. *Pain, 41,* 295-301.

Tait, R. C., Pollard, C. A., Margolis, R. B., Duckro, P. N., & Krause, S. J. The pain disability index: Psychometric and validity data. *Archives of Physical Medicine and Rehabilitation, 68*, 438-441.

Tan, Tjiauw-ling; et al (1984). Biopsychobehavioral correlates of insomnia: IV. Diagnosis based on DSM-III. *American Journal of Psychiatry, 141*, 357-362.

Tasto, D. L. (1977). Self-report schedules and inventories. In A. Ciminero, K. Calhoun, & H. Adams (Eds.), Handbook of behavioral assessment (pp. 153-193). New York: Wiley.

Taub, A. (1973). Relief of postherpetic neuralgia with psychotropic drugs. *Journal of Neurosurgery, 39*, 235 – 239.

Taub, A., & Collins, W. F. (1974). Observations on the treatment of denervation dysesthesia with psychotropic drugs: Postherpetic neuralgia, anesthesia, dolorossa, peripheral neuropathy. *Advances in Neurology, 4*, 309 – 315.

Tayer, W. G., Nicassio, P. M., Radojevic, V., & Krall, T. (1996). Pain and helplessness as correlates of depression in systemic lupus erythematosus. *British Journal of Health Psychology, 1*, 253-262.

Taylor, A., Lorentzen, L., & Blank, M. (1990). Psychologic distress of chronic pain sufferers and their spouses. *Journal of Pain and Symptom Management, 5*, 6-10.

Taylor, J. A. (1953). A personality scale of manifest anxiety. *Journal of Abnormal and Social Psychology, 48*, 285-290.

Taylor, C. B., Sallis, J. F., & Needle, R. (1985). The relation of physical activity and exercise to mental health. *Public Health Reports, 100*, 195-202.

Tellenbach, H. (1983). *Melancholie*. Berlin: Springer.

Temoshok, L. & Dreher, H. (1993). *The Type C connection: The mind-body link to cancer and your health*. New York: Plume.

Tennant, C., Mihailidou, A., Smith, A., Smith, R., Kellow, J., Jones, M., Hunyor, S., Lorang, M., & Hoschl, R. (1994).

Psychological symptom profiles in patients with chest pain. *Journal of Psychosomatic Research, 38,* 365-371.

Thomas, M. R., & Roy, R. (1999). *The changing nature of pain complaints over the lifespan.* New York: Plenum Press.

Tkachuk, G. A., & Martin, G. L. (1999). Exercise therapy for patients with psychiatric disorders: Research and clinical implications. *Professional Psychology: Research & Practice, 30,* 275-282.

Tomkins, S. S. (1991). *Affect, imagery, and consciousness.Vol. 3. The negative affects: anger and fear.* New York: Springer.

Torgerson, W. S., & BenDebba, M. (1983). The structure of pain descriptors. In R. Melzack (Ed.). *Pain measurement and assessment* (pp. 49-54). New York: Raven Press.

Towery, S., & Fernandez, E. (1996). Reclassification and rescaling of McGill Pain Questionnaire verbal descriptors of pain sensation: A replication. *The Clinical Journal of Pain, 12,* 270-276.

Tracey, T. J., & Kokotovic, A. M. (1989). Factor structure of the Working Alliance Inventory. *Psychological Assessment, 1,* 207-210.

Traskman-Bendz, L., Ekman, R., Regnell, G., & Ohman, R. (1992). HPA-related CSF neuropeptides in suicide attempters. *European Neuropsychoplarmacology, 2,* 99-106.

Tschannen, T. A., Duckro, P. N., Margolis, R. B. & Tomazic, T. J. (1992). The relationship of anger, depression, and perceived disability among headache patients. *Headache, 32,* 501-503.

Turk, D. C. (1996). Cognitive factors in chronic pain and disability. In K. D. Craig & K. Dobson (Eds.), *State of the art in cognitive/behavioral therapy* (pp. 83-115) Beverly Hills, CA: Sage.

Turk, D. C. & Fernandez, E. (1990). On the putative uniqueness of cancer pain: Do psychological principles apply? *Behaviour Research and Therapy, 28,* 1-13.

Turk, D. C., & Fernandez, E. (1995). Personality assessment and the Minnesota Multiphasic Personality Inventory in chronic pain. *The Pain Forum, 4*, 104-107.

Turk, D. C., & Okifuji, A. (1994). Detecting depression in chronic pain patients: adequacy of self-reports. *Behavior Research and Therapy, 32*, 9-16.

Turk, D. C., & Okifuji, A. (1997). Evaluating the role of physical, operant, cognitive, and affective factors in the pain behaviors of chronic pain patients. *Behavior Modification, 21,* 259-280.

Turk, D. C., Rudy, T. E., & Salovey, P. (1985). The McGill Pain Questionnaire reconsidered: Confirming the factor structure and examining appropriate uses. *Pain, 21*, 386-397.

Turnbull, F. (1979). The nature of pain that may accompany cancer of the lung. *Pain, 7,* 371-375.

Turner, J. A., & Romano, J. M. (1984). Self-report screening measures for depression in chronic pain patients. *Journal of Clinical Psychology, 40*, 909 - 913.

Turner, J. A., & Jensen, M. P. (1993). Efficacy of cognitive therapy for chronic low back pain. *Pain, 52*, 169-177.

Turner, R. J., & Noh, S. (1988). Physical disability and depression: a longitudinal analysis. *Journal of Health and Social Behavior, 29*, 23-37.

Tyber, M. A. (1974). Treatment of the painful shoulder syndrome with amitryptiline and lithium carbonate. *Canadian Medical Association Journal, 111*, 137-140.

Urban, B. J., France, R. D., Bissette, G., Spielman, F. J., & Nemeroff, C. B. (1988). Alterations in cerebrospinal fluid concentrations of somatostatin-like immunoreactivity in chronic pain patients. *Pain, 33,* 169-172.

Van Houdenhove, B., & Knapen, P. (1986). Academisch Psychiatrisch Ctr Salve Mater, Lovenjoel, Belgium De relatie tussen chronische pijn en depressie: II. Therapeutische aspecten. /The relationship between chronic pain and depression: II. Therapeutic aspects. *Tijdschrift voor Psychiatrie, 28,* 145-165.

Van Houdenhove, B., Vestraeten, D., Onghena, P., & de Cuyper, H. (1992). Chronic idiopathic pain, mianserin and "masked" depression. *Psychotherapy & Psychosomatics, 58,* 46-53.

Van Kempen, G. M., Zitman, F. G., Linssen, A. C., & Edelbroek, P. M. (1992). Biochemical measures in patients with a somatoform pain disorder, before, during, and after treatment with amitriptyline with or without flupentixol. *Biological Psychiatry, 31,* 670-680.

Van Peski-Oosterbaan, A. S., Spinhoven, P., van Rood, Y., Van der Does, A. J., Willem, B., & Albert J. V. (1997). Cognitive behavioural therapy for unexplained non-cardiac chest pain: A pilot study. *Behavioural & Cognitive Psychotherapy, 25,* 339-350.

VanDyck, R., Zitman, F. G., Linssen, A. C., Spinhoven, P. (1991). Autogenic training and future oriented hypnotic imagery in the treatment of tension headache: Outcome and process. *International Journal of Clinical & Experimental Hypnosis, 39,* 6-23.

Varni, J. W., Rapoff, M. A., Waldron, S. A., Gragg, R. A., et al. (1996). Chronic pain and emotional distress in children and adolescents. *Journal of Developmental & Behavioral Pediatrics, 17,* 154-161.

Vassend, O. (1993). Anxiety, pain and discomfort associated with dental treatment. *Behaviour Research & Therapy, 31,* 659-666.

Vassend, O., Krogstad, B. S., & Dahl, B. L. (1995). Negative affectivity, somatic complaints, and symptoms of temporomandibular disorders. *Journal of Psychosomatic Research, 39,* 889-899.

Velikova, G., Selby, P. J., Snaith, P. R., & Kirby, P. G. (1995). The relationship of cancer pain to anxiety. *Psychotherapy & Psychosomatics, 63,* 181-184.

Verma, S., & Gallagher, R. M. (2000). Evaluating and treating co-morbid pain and depression. *International Review of Psychiatry, 12*, 103-114.

Villarreal, S. S. (1995). A comparative study of selected patient variables as risk factors in hospitalization for chronic headache. *Headache, 35*, 349-354.

Vimpari, S. S., Knuutila, M. L., Sakki, T. K., & Kivela, S. L. (1995). Depressive symptoms associated with symptoms of the temporamandibular joint pain and dysfunction syndrome. *Psychosomatic Medicine, 57*, 437-444.

Viney, L. (1986). Expression of positive emotion by people who are physically ill: Is it evidence of defending or coping? *Journal of Psychosomatic Research, 30*, 27-34.

Violon, A. (1980). The onset of facial pain: A psychological study. *Psychotherapy & Psychosomatics, 34*, 11-16.

Vittengl, J. R.; Clark, L. A., Owen-Salters, E., Gatchel, R. J. (1999). Diagnostic change and personality stability following functional restoration treatment in chronic low back pain patients. *Assessment, 6*, 79-91.

von Baeyer, C. L., Carlson, G., & Webb, L. (1997). Underprediction of pain in children undergoing ear piercing. *Behaviour Research & Therapy, 35*, 399-404.

von Brauchitsch, H. (1975). Masked depression and pain. *Biological Psychology Bulletin, 4*, 72-80.

von Frey, M. (1896). Untersuchungen uber die Sinnesfunctionen der menschlichen Haut. Druckempfinding und Schmerz, Abh. Math.-phys. Class Konigl. Sachsischen *Gesellschaft der Wissenschaften, 23*, 175-264.

von Knorring, L. (1978). An experimental study of visual average evoked responses (V, AER), and pain measures (PM) in patients with depressive disorders. *Biological Psychology, 6*, 27-38.

von Knorring, L. (1989) The pathogenesis of chronic pain syndromes. *Nordisk Psykiatrisk Tidsskrift, 43(Suppl. 20),* 35-41.

von Knorring, L., & Ekselius, L. (1994). Idiopathic pain and depression. *Quality of Life Research: An International Journal of Quality of Life Aspects of Treatment, Care & Rehabilitation, 3*, S57-S68.

von Knorring, L., & Espvall, M. (1974). Experimentally induced pain in patients with depressive disorders. *Acta Psychiatrica Scandinavica, Suppl., 255*, 121-133.

von Knorring, L., Almay, B.G. L., & Johansson, F. (1987). Personality traits in patients with idiopathic pain disorder. *Acta Psychiatry Scand, 76*, 490-498.

von Knorring, L., Perris, C., Eisemann, M., Eriksson, U., & Perris, H. (1983). Pain as a symptom in depressive disorders: I. Relationship to diagnostic subgroup and depressive symptomatology. *Pain, 15,* 19-26.

von Knorring, L., Perris, C., Eisemann, M., & Eriksson, U. (1989). Pain as a symptom in depressive disorders: Relationship to social background factors. *The European Journal of Psychiatry, 3*, 99-104.

von Korff, M., Dworkin, S. F., le Resche, L., & Kruger, A. (1988). An epidemiologic comparison of pain complaints. *Pain, 32*, 173-183.

von Korff, M., Dworkin, S. F., le Resche, L., & Kruger, A. (1988). An epidemiologic comparison of pain complaints. *Source Pain, 32*, 173-183.

Waddell, G., Newton, M., Henderson, I., Somerville, D., & Main, C.J. (1993). A Fear-Avoidance Beliefs Questionnaire (FABQ) and the role of fear-avoidance beliefs in chronic low back pain and disability. *Pain, 52*, 157-168.

Wade, D. T., Leigh-Smith, J., & Hewer, R. A. (1987). Depressed mood after stroke: A community study of its frequency. *British Journal of Psychiatry, 151*, 200-205.

Wade, J. B., Price, D. D., Hamer, R. M., Schwartz, S. M., & Hart, R. P. (1990). An emotional component analysis of chronic pain. *Pain, 40*, 303-310.

Walker, E., Katon, W., Harrop-Griffiths, J., Holm, L. et al (1988). Relationship of chronic pelvic pain to psychiatric diagnoses and childhood sexual abuse. *American Journal of Psychiatry, 145,* 75-80.

Wall, V. J., & Womack, W. (1989). Hypnotic versus active cognitive strategies for alleviation of procedural distress in pediatric oncology patients. *American Journal of Clinical Hypnosis, 31,* 181-191.

Wallace, L. M. (1986). Pre-operative state anxiety as a mediator of psychological adjustment to and recovery from surgery. *British Journal of Medical Psychology, 59,* 253-261.

Wallace, L. M. (1985). Surgical patients' expectations of pain and discomfort: Does accuracy of expectations minimize post-surgical pain and distress? *Pain, 22,* 363-373.

Wallace, L. M. (1987). Trait anxiety as a predictor of adjustment to and recovery from surgery. *British Journal of Clinical Psychology, 26,* 73-74.

Wallston, K. A., Wallston, B. S., & DeVellis, R. (1978). Development of the Multidimensional Health Locus of Control (MHLC) scales. *Health Education Monographs, 6,* 160-170.

Ward, N. G., Bloom, V. L., & Friedel, R. O. (1979). The effectiveness of tricyclic antidepressants in the treatment of coexisting pain and depression. *Pain, 14,* 331-341.

Ward, N. G., Bloom, V. L., Dworkin, S., Fawcett, J., Narasimhachari, N., & Friedel, R.O. (1982). Psychobiological markers in coexisting pain and depression: Toward a unified theory. *Journal of Clinical Psychiatry, 43,* 32-39.

Ward, N. G., Turner, J. A., Ready, B., & Bigos, S. J. (1992). Chronic pain, depression, and the dexamethasone suppression test. *Pain, 48,* 331-338.

Wardle, J. (1987). Psychological management of anxiety and pain during dental treatment. *Journal of Psychosomatic Research, l 27,* 399-402

Wardle, J. (1982). Fear of dentistry. *British Journal of Medical Psychology, 155,* 119-126.

Ware, J. E., Snow, K. K., Kosinski, M., & Gandek, B. (1993). *SF-36 Health Survey: Manual and interpretation guide.* Boston: The Health Institute, New England Medical Center.

Watson, C. P., Evans, R. J., & Reed, K., et al (1982). Amitriptyline versus placebo in postherpetic neuraligic. *Neurology, 32,* 671 – 673.

Watson, C. P., Evans, R. J., Reed, K., Merskey, H., Goldsmith, L., & Warsh, J. (1982). Amitriptyline versus placebo in postherpetic neuralgia. *Neurology, 32,* 671-673.

Weickgenant, A. L., Slater, M. A., Patterson, T. L., Atkinson, J. H., Grant, I., & Garfin, S. R. (1993). Coping activities in chronic low back pain: relationship with depression. *Pain, 53,* 95-103.

Weiner, B. (1985). An attributional theory of achievement, motivation and emotion. *Psychological Review, 92,* 548-573.

Weiner, D. J. (1999). *Beyond talk therapy: Using movement and expressive techniques in clinical practice.* Washington, D.C.: American Psychological Association.

Weisenberg, M. (1975). *Pain: Clinical and experimental perspectives.* Mosby. St. Louis, MO.

Weisenberg, M. et al (1985). Subject versus experimenter control in the reaction to pain. *Pain, 23,* 187-200.

Wells, J. K., Howard, G. S., Nowlin, W. F., & Vargas, M. J. (1986). Presurgical anxiety and postsurgical pain and adjustment: Effects of a stress inoculation procedure. *Journal of Consulting & Clinical Psychology, 54,* 831-835.

Wells, K. B., Golding, J. M., & Burnham, M. A. (1988). Psychiatric disorder in a sample of the general population with and without chronic medical conditions. *American Journal of Psychiatry, 145,* 976-981.

Wells, K. B., Golding, J. M., & Burnham, M. A. (1989). Affective, substance use, and anxiety diorders in persons with arthritis, diabetes, heart disease, high blood pressure,or chronic lung conditions. *General Hospital Psychiatry*, *11*, 320-327.

Wells, K. B., Stewart, A., Hays, R. D., Burnam, M. A., Rogers, W., Daniels, M., Berry, S., Greenfield, S., & Ware, J. (1989). The functioning and well-being of depressed patients: Results from the Medical Outcomes Study. *Journal of the American Medical Association*, *262*, 914 - 919.

Wertheimer, M. (1923). Untersuchungen zur Lehre von der Gestalt, II. *Psychologische Forschung*, *4*, 301-350.

Westra, H. A., & Stewart, S. H. (2002). As-needed use of benzodiazepines in managing clinical anxiety: incidence and implications. *Current Pharmaceutical Design*, *8*, 59-74.

Westwell, P., & Johnson, N. F. (1988). A comparison of pain vocabulary and affective symptoms in patients with malignant and non-malignant disorders. *Medical Science Research*, *16*, 583-584.

Widerstroem, E. G., Aslund, P. G., Gustafsson, L. E., Mannheimer, C., et al (1982). Relations between experimentally induced tooth pain threshold changes, psychometrics and clinical pain relief following TENS: A retrospective study in patients with long-lasting pain. *Pain*, *51*, 281-287.

Widlocher, D. J. (1983). Psychomotor retardation: Clinical, theoretical, and psychometric aspects. *Psychiatric Clinics of North America*, *6*, 27– 40.

Widmer, R. B., & Cadoret, R. J. (1978). Depression in primary care: changes in pattern of patient visits and complaints during a developing depression. *Journal of Family Practice*, *7*, 293-302.

Williams, A. C. (1998). Depression in chronic pain: Mistaken models, missed opportunities. *Scandinavian Journal of Behaviour Therapy*, *27*, 61-80 .

Williams, A. C., & Richardson, P. H. (1993). What does the BDI measure in chronic pain? *Pain*, *55*, 259-266.

Williams, J. B. W., & Spitzer, R. L. (1982). Idiopathic pain disorder: A critique of pain-prone disorder and a proposal for a revision an the DSM-III category psychogenic pain disorder. *Journal of Nervous and Mental Disease, 170,* 415-419.

Wilson, W. P.; Blazer, D. G.; Nashold, B. S. (1976). Observations on pain and suffering. *Psychosomatics, 17,* 73-76.

Wittkower, E. D. & Warnes, H. (Eds.) (1984). *Psychosomatic medicine: Its clinical applications.* New York: Harper & Row.

Woodforde, J. M., & Merskey, H. (1972). Personality traits of patients with chronic pain. *Journal of Psychosomatic Research, 16,* 167-172.

Woodworth, R. S. (1918). *Dynamic psychology.* New York: Columbia University Press.

Worthington, J. J., Pollack, M. H., Otto, M. W., Gould, R. A., et al (1997). Panic disorder in emergency ward patients with chest pain. *Journal of Nervous & Mental Disease, 185,* 274-276.

Yensen, R. (1988). Helping at the edges of life: Perspectives of a psychedelic therapist. *Journal of Near-Death Studies, 6,* 149-161.

Yilmaz, A., & Weiss, M. G. (2000). Cultural formulation: Depression and back pain in a young male Turkish immigrant in Basel, Switzerland. *Culture, Medicine & Psychiatry, 24,* 259-272.

Young, Jeffrey E. (1999). *Cognitive therapy for personality disorders: A schema-focused approach* (3rd ed.). Sarasota, FL: Professional Resource Press/Professional Resource Exchange, Inc.

Young, L., & Humphrey, M. (1985). Cognitive methods of preparing women for hysterectomy: Does a booklet help? *British Journal of Clinical Psychology, 24,* 303-304.

Zelin, M. L., Adler, G., & Myerson, P. G. (1972). Anger self-report: An objective questionnaire for the measurement of aggression. *Journal of Consulting and Clinical Psychology*, *39*, 340.

Zeltzer, L., & LeBaron, S. (1986). Assessment of acute pain and anxiety and chemotherapy-related nausea and vomiting in children and adolescents. *Hospice Journal*, *2*, 75-98.

Ziegler, D. K., Rhodes, R. J., & Hassanein, R. S. (1978). Association of psychological measurements of anxiety and depression with headache history in a non-child poplation. *Research and Clinical Studies on Headache*, *6*, 123-135.

Zigmond, A. S., & Snaith, R. P. (1983). The hospital anxiety and depression scale. *Acta Psychiatrica Scand.*, *67*, 361-370.

Zimmermann-Tansella, C., Dolcetta, G., Azzini, V., Zacche, G., Bertagni, P., Siani, R., & Tansella, M. (1979). Preparation courses for childbirth in primipara: A comparison. *Journal of Psychosomatic Research*, *23*, 227-233.

Zuckerman, M., Kolin, E. A., Price, L., & Zoob, I. (1964). Development of a sensation-seeking scale. *Journal of Consulting Psychology*, *6*, 477-482.

Zung, W. W. K. (1965). A self-rating depression scale. *Archives of General Psychiatry*, *12*, 63-65.

Index